AF782747

Quality Patient Care in Hospitals

Quality Patient Care in Hospitals

Dr Dennis Green

BSi
Business Information

Dedication

This book is dedicated to:

my wife, Margaret

my three daughters and three sons-in-law

Alison and John

Helen and Anthony

Caroline and Karl

and my eight grandchildren

Thomas, Lucy, Sophie and Emily, Harriet and Alexander, Jessica and Rebecca

First published in the UK in 2005
by
BSI
389 Chiswick High Road
London W4 4AL

© British Standards Institution 2005

All rights reserved. Except as permitted under the Copyright, Designs and Patents Act 1988, no part of this publication may be reproduced, stored in a retrieval system or transmitted in any form or by any means – electronic, photocopying, recording or otherwise – without prior permission in writing from the publisher.

Whilst every care has been taken in developing and compiling this publication, BSI accepts no liability for any loss or damage caused, arising directly or indirectly in connection with reliance on its contents except to the extent that such liability may not be excluded in law.

The right of Dennis Green to be identified as the author of this Work has been asserted by him in accordance with sections 77 and 78 of the Copyright, Designs and Patents Act 1988.

Typeset in Great Britain by Typobatics Ltd

Printed in Great Britain by The Charlesworth Group

British Library Cataloguing in Publication Data

A catalogue record for this book is available from the British Library

ISBN 0 580 45646 3

Table of Contents

Preface

Nobody can be more passionate than me about wanting National Health Service (NHS) hospitals to be among the best hospitals in the world for diagnosing and treating patients. Shortly after I was appointed the assistant regional physicist in the Department of Clinical Physics and Bio-Engineering in the Glasgow Health Board (the biggest department of its kind in the world at the time). I became clinically involved with pacemaker patients in several hospitals in and around Glasgow, at operation, at pacemaker clinics and at post-mortems. In due course the number of pacemaker patients exceeded 1,000. I believe the service that was provided for such patients was second to none – and many clinicians in the rest of the world recognized this fact. Patients with suspected heart problems were diagnosed quickly, surgery followed within days and any serious life threatening cases were admitted immediately and patients were made safe with an external pacemaker, prior to surgery. Within a matter of days, most patients returned home to live a virtually normal life. At pacemaker follow-up clinics the patients were so very grateful and they showed this by their comments and the delight on their faces. Often, I went home feeling so proud that I had made a small contribution to the well-being and happiness of so many patients fitted with pacemakers in the Glasgow region. I also realized that it was indeed a great privilege to be working so closely with so many medical and surgical colleagues in the Glasgow hospitals, who treated me as a professional in my own right. Today, millions of people around the world now benefit from having a pacemaker implanted.

I imagine that many other specialties in diagnosis and treatment have excelled in our NHS hospitals over the years and many other millions of patients must be grateful for the diagnosis and treatment they have received. Moreover, progress continues year on year as medical science and technology advance. Yet, in spite of all such advances, there is a general perception that all is not well with our NHS hospitals. Things are not as good as they ought to be. After all these years, successive governments have failed in their attempts to meet the needs of so many patients and many different excuses have been given. Yet few, if any, experts in the field seem to have suggested that better management might improve the situation in a relatively short time. I believe that application of the ISO 9001 quality management system standard to our hospitals would result in real improvements at relatively little cost and within a short period of time.

The ISO 9001 quality management system standard was published in December 2000. It was the culmination of several years' work by the international Technical Committee 176 of the International Organization for Standardization (ISO), which had met at regular intervals following the publication of the last revision of the standard in 1994. The revision of standards is a routine procedure and the committees responsible always consider any feedback from users of an existing standard. In the case of ISO 9001:2000, it replaced three of the 1994 standards (9001, 9002 and 9003). The draft international standard was circulated widely for comments. The end result is not a perfect revised standard, but there is general agreement that ISO 9001:2000 is an improvement on its precursors.

The latest data published in September 2004, shows that by the end of 2003, over half a million ISO 9000 certificates (old and new versions) had been awarded in well over 100 countries [1].

ISO 9001 is applicable to both large and small organizations. What is surprising is that no NHS hospital, as far as I am aware, has taken up the challenge of trying to achieve accredited certification to ISO 9001. Many private hospitals have done so.

ISO 9001 is about striving at all times to get things right and to do things better. It is not about being perfect: all of us make mistakes occasionally but we can try and reduce the occurrences of adverse events, untoward incidents, system failures or human error and introduce actions that reduce the likelihood of such events happening again.

ISO 9001 is about putting top management in control. It is also about openness, integrity and accountability. These are the core requirements of corporate governance and indeed the basis of clinical audit (see Appendix 2). Chief executives are now responsible for reporting on clinical governance. All the other initiatives in the care of patients, such as the Commission for Healthcare Audit and Inspection (CHAI) (see Appendix 3), would benefit from the introduction of ISO 9001 to a hospital.

A minimum amount of documentation is required. Once the basic requirements have been met, senior staff can decide what documentation is required. All documentation and records must be properly controlled. ISO 9001 is a process-based management system standard and a number of process diagrams are included. These encourage logical thinking, the integration of the actions of everyone and minimum amounts of paperwork.

Chapter 9 addresses clause 7.3, design and development, and in particular its application to hospitals. Appendix 1 includes, by way of example, the six mandatory procedures required by the standard.

If a hospital implemented an ISO 9001 quality management system, it would be required to conduct its own internal audits. This requirement must be considered in a positive manner. Nobody is exempt from internal auditing, however senior. Auditors have to be trained in internal auditing and the collection of objective evidence. In the case of ISO 9001, nobody can audit their own work. Clinical audits and their correlation with ISO 9001 auditing are discussed in Chapter 10. Chapter 11 gives guideline audit questions for both ISO 9001 and for those attempting to improve their clinical auditing skills.

A number of hospital departments have already achieved accreditation to ISO 9001. I have audited a number of hospital departments on behalf of accredited certification bodies. However, as stated above, the true benefits will accrue to a hospital only when the entire hospital has achieved accredited certification. I am confident that once the first hospital has achieved accredited certification, other hospitals will want to follow.

It would be impossible to thank personally all of those who have made the writing of this book possible. Much of the book is based on my experience as an auditor, mainly auditing against the quality management standard on behalf of certification bodies. I should like to express my thanks to these certification bodies, which have provided me with many opportunities for third-party auditing. I should also like to thank the people in the many organizations that I have subjected to the rigours of third-party auditing. All the people that I have met at different levels within such organizations have, without exception, received me kindly and enabled me to carry out my duties. Without such acceptance, auditing would have become an unwelcome task and one that I would have abandoned a long time ago.

Acknowledgement

I am indebted to Dr Peter B. Savege, lately primary care adviser to Barnet, Enfield and Haringey Health Authority for carefully reading the text of this book at its various stages of preparation and for making extremely useful criticisms and corrections.

Chapter 1: General introduction

This book was prompted by my realization that no British National Health Service (NHS) hospital, as far as I'm aware, has achieved accredited certification to the quality management systems standard, ISO 9001. There may be many reasons for this, but the main reason is probably that the other demands made on hospitals by government departments have had to be given greater priority. However, now that government priorities have been or are being addressed after the provision of large amounts of money to the NHS, perhaps more attention will be given to better management of complex organizations such as hospitals. Some hospital departments have achieved certification to the standard: these have been the more scientifically based departments in hospitals. However, the real benefits from accredited certification will accrue to a hospital only when the entire hospital is functioning under the ethos and requirements of the standard. ISO 9001 should put top management in better control with everyone in a hospital working together for the benefit of patients.

Some private hospitals in the UK, which are much smaller than NHS hospitals, have already achieved accredited certification. The introduction of a number of private treatment centres into the British NHS will provide further opportunities for the application of the standard. These private treatment centres will provide specialist surgery for cataracts, hip and knee replacements, hernia and other day surgery, free at the point of need and funded by the government. These treatment centres will not have their planned operations delayed by any other unplanned demands such as emergency admissions that sometimes interrupt planned operations in NHS hospitals.

ISO 9001 is an international standard that can be taken up by hospitals worldwide.

British National Health Service (NHS) hospitals

The British NHS has stood as a cornerstone of all political parties since it was launched in 1948 after the end of the Second World War. Many new hospitals have been built over the last half century. There are now more doctors and supporting staff than ever before. Developments in medical science and modern technology have enabled more and more patients to gain an improved quality of life than was conceivable when the NHS was launched. Moreover, as lifespan has steadily increased over the last half century, more and more elderly people have been treated successfully so that they have a quality of life that was not possible for their forebears. This record of progress in alleviating suffering and improving the quality of life of patients of all ages has proved to be sustainable.

More government money is being allocated to the NHS. During the tax year 2004–2005 over £80 billion will be spent on the NHS; this is planned to increase in real terms to the order of £100 billion by 2007–2008. The NHS employs over a million people making it one of the biggest employers in Europe. The NHS provides an excellent accident and emergency service. However, patients may have to wait a long time before they are treated. Many patients attend hospitals each year for diagnosis and treatment, and the overwhelming majority are very grateful for the treatment they receive. Nevertheless, there is a general perception that the NHS is failing to meet expectations in many ways. For instance, at the time of writing, about one million patients are waiting to be admitted to NHS hospitals for planned routine operations. As a consequence of this and other shortcomings, a lot of people have to suffer unnecessarily.

Many reasons have been given for the failure of the NHS to meet people's expectations. There have been repeated demands for more money, more doctors, more nurses, more support staff, better hospital buildings and improved technology. Surprisingly, one has rarely heard demands for better management of hospitals. Indeed, in the early days of the NHS, there was little management of hospitals as we know it today.

In the 1970s the Greater Glasgow Health Board was reorganized. The author recalls being told that as a result of the reorganization 94 committees of the Greater Glasgow Health Board were created. It prompted the author to say to the Secretary of the Board (the Chief Non-medical Officer) that what the Health Board needed, above all else, was a single manager: in effect a chief executive, medically qualified or otherwise, to manage all the hospitals in the vicinity of Glasgow. Their salary would have to be high in order to recruit one of the best people available for such an important task.

Later on when managers were introduced into NHS hospitals, they were given responsibility for financial control of the hospitals. In 2002, they were given additional responsibility for reporting on clinical governance. It seemed that government had, at last, come to realize the importance of first-class management of our hospitals. Now that we have chief executives and more managers in place, the question needs to be asked whether they are of the right calibre and, more importantly, whether they are in control. Evidently they are not always in control, for several have had their employment terminated in recent times for poor performance and a number have resigned.

All of these changes, in terms of additional resources and the introduction of chief executives, provide exceptional opportunities to improve the NHS.

A number of other important changes have also taken place. For instance, for the first time, steps have been taken in recent years to monitor systematically the performance of clinicians. Medical audit and clinical audit are two such initiatives. These, together with Sir Adrian Cadbury's earlier report on Corporate Governance [2], led to the concept of clinical governance (see Appendix 2). Perhaps even more significant are the many initiatives that have been established to focus on the care of patients in hospitals (see Appendix 3). These include:

The National Institute for Clinical Excellence (NICE);

National Service Frameworks (NSFs);

Patient Advice and Liaison Services (PALS);

The Independent Complaints Advocacy Service (ICAS);

The Patients' and Public Involvement Forums (PPIs);

The National Patient Safety Agency (NPSA);

National Surveys of Patient and User Experience;

The Commission for Health Improvement (CHI).

A new health care commission was established on 1 April 2004 for England and Wales with a remit to inspect NHS, private and voluntary health care facilities. The legal name of the new health care commission is the Commission for Healthcare Audit and Inspection. CHAI has taken over all the former work of the Commission for Health Improvement (CHI), the NHS 'value for money' work of the Audit Commission, the Mental Health Act Commission (MHAC), and the independent health care work of the former National Care Standards Commission (NCSC), which was responsible for the oversight of private health care. The National Care Standards Commission was superseded on 1 April 2004 by the Commission for Social Care Inspection (CSCI).

The new inspectorate (CHAI) will assess the performance of every part of the NHS. Most importantly, it will be independent of government and independent of the NHS.

The inspectorate will report annually to parliament on the performance of the NHS and the uses to which its resources have been put. More specifically it intends to:

- encourage improvement in the quality and effectiveness of care and in the economy and efficiency of its provision;
- inspect the management, provision and quality of health care services and track where, and how well, public resources are being used;
- carry out investigations into serious service failures;
- report serious concerns about the quality of public services to the Secretary of State;
- publish annual performance ratings for all NHS organizations and produce annual reports to parliament on the state of health care;
- collaborate with other relevant organizations including the Commission for Social Care Inspection (CSCI);
- carry out an independent review function for NHS complaints.

The CHAI website can be located at www.chai.org.uk.

Hospitals are complex organizations. They are complex because they are usually large organizations that employ a lot of people and have a lot of specialized equipment. Moreover, they usually have a large number of highly qualified professional people, many of whom are not used to being managed at all, particularly by managers not of their own profession. Traditionally, doctors have always worked independently. However, their individual clinical independence has been eroded by the gradual, but continual, growth of evidence-based medicine. Absolute clinical freedom is not possible now, although appropriate clinical freedom will continue under the surveillance of clinical governance and bodies such as CHAI.

Hospitals also have to manage the experiences of thousands of patients: their routine admissions to the hospital, the time that they spend in hospital, their diagnosis and possible treatment, and the problems of discharge, including bed blocking. A large number of patients also attend hospital as day-patients and as out-patients. In addition, there are emergency admissions to hospitals often via accident and emergency departments.

It is very important that the resources allocated to the NHS are managed well. If the NHS is to become a service that provides quality patient care it needs the best top management that can be found. It is a little surprising that, in spite of the other priorities referred to earlier, NHS hospitals have failed to take up ISO 9001 to maintain and continually improve their performance by means of a quality management system.

The international standard ISO 9001:2000

ISO 9001:2000 has its origins in military standards going back to an American military standard first published in 1959. The first non-military standard was the British standard BS 5750:1979. The International Organization for Standardization (ISO) based in Switzerland later became involved and the first international quality systems standard was published in 1987. These standards were again revised by ISO in 1994. The latest revision occurred in December 2000 with the publication of the quality management systems standard, ISO 9001:2000. These standards have been used by all kinds of organizations, such as manufacturers, service industries and professional bodies.

The purpose of ISO 9001 is to make all kinds of organizations more efficient, with the prime focus on achieving customer satisfaction. When the standard is applied to a hospital, the prime focus is on achieving patient satisfaction. Any organization that achieves customer satisfaction gains two more important benefits. First, such organizations are happier organizations in that everyone takes a better interest and pride in their work. Second, and if the organization is striving for profits, there is a likelihood that an efficient organization will make more profit than an inefficient one. Public service organizations, such as NHS hospitals, do not exist to make profits, but any highly organized body is likely to be more efficient and cost effective.

The format of the revised standard is different from its precursors. There are only five requirement clauses to be addressed in ISO 9001 and only six procedures are mandatory. Otherwise a hospital can decide what documentation is required for it to function in an efficient manner.

The standard does not require staff to be perfect. Nevertheless, ISO 9001 encourages management and employees to strive to achieve perfection. The more complex an organization is the more difficult it is for managers and individuals to achieve such an objective.

The revised standard is very different from its precursors in one very important way. It is not intended that the quality management system should sit alongside the processes of the organization and interrupt or interfere with those processes as and when indicated by the different clauses of ISO 9001. On the contrary, a quality management system is intended to become so closely integrated with the processes of an organization that the two become inseparable.

There will be some activities in a hospital, for instance sterilization of surgical instruments, which can stand alone and be checked in isolation from any major hospital processes involving surgery. Clause 7.5.2 of ISO 9001 deals with validation of processes for production and service provision. The particular example of sterilization is an essential part of surgical processes, although the validation process is done outside the operating theatre. The same is true of similar activities that are essential to the success of surgical processes. The quality management system of the hospital will recognize the importance of all such activities, but the main focus will be on integrating all such support processes into several major surgical processes.

In Chapter 3, a number of major hospital processes have been depicted by process diagrams. The back-up essential support processes, such as sterilization of surgical instruments, are referred to as lower-level processes.

It soon becomes evident that certification to ISO 9001 is not a 'tick-box' process, in which each tick box is isolated from other clauses of the standard. An integrated approach is required in which the focus is on both the organization's quality management system and the major processes for which the organization exists. Top management must develop a quality management system based on the requirements of the standard that will enable it to organize its processes better. There should be a continuing desire to achieve improvements in the ways in which the organization functions, and the onus is on top management to continually improve the effectiveness of the quality management system and, thereby, the overall effectiveness of all its activities.

The use of process diagrams (or flow charts) significantly reduces the amount of text required and enables an organization to rationalize its activities more easily. Every organization has at least one major process: some have many major processes.

Organizations seeking certification against the requirements of ISO 9001 are audited by professionally qualified auditors. Such auditors are commissioned by certification bodies, which in turn are scrutinized by national bodies. In the UK, this body is the United Kingdom Accreditation Service (UKAS). UKAS itself is scrutinized by an external organization to ensure that it too is complying with international agreements for such bodies. Thus, every effort is made to ensure that any accredited certifications are worthy of the name and are awarded against the same international criteria.

Clinical audits

Clinical audit emerged in 1993 shortly after the concepts of corporate governance were first enunciated. These concepts were first introduced into the NHS under the title of Clinical Governance in 1997 (see Appendix 2). The Commission for Health Improvement (CHI), created in 2000, took over the responsibility for clinical governance (Appendix 3). More recently, CHI became responsible for directing clinical audits in hospitals. CHAI will now assume this role. Clinical audits are discussed in more detail in Appendix 2. Suffice it to say at this stage that there are similarities between ISO 9001 audits and clinical audits. Any hospital that has excelled in clinical audits by the independent inspectorate should consider seeking accredited certification to ISO 9001, as the findings of clinical audit could well be accepted, subject to verification, by a certification body as part of the greater picture of first-class management control of all the activities that take place within a hospital.

Terminology

The ISO 9001 Quality Management Systems standard is a generic document that refers throughout to product, although the reader of the standard is asked to interpret 'product' as 'product or service', or both, as is appropriate.

The product of a hospital

Before interpreting the standard for application to hospitals, it is necessary to clarify what is meant by the product of a hospital. In all hospitals, staff are striving to add value to the quality of life of all patients. In other words, the product of hospitals is the 'improved quality of life', where possible, of patients that result from all the activities that take place within the hospital. It is a somewhat cumbersome definition, but it helps to interpret the standard for application to hospitals.

The definition given for the product of a hospital has some analogy with the products of a manufacturer. The manufacturer will add value to materials or parts (or both) to improve the overall output. This analogy may not be perfect, but the concept of the 'improved quality of life' of patients as being the product of a hospital is a useful one and helps to avoid muddled thinking over product and services in applying ISO 9001 to hospitals.

The services of a hospital

There is no doubt about what is meant by services in the context of a hospital. The services provided are all the clinical and other activities that are provided for the ultimate benefit of patients, whether they are of direct or indirect benefit to patients.

Quality

It is important to understand what is meant by the word quality when used in connection with hospitals. The word 'quality' is used in all kinds of situations: such as quality products, quality services and quality value. Politicians frequently talk about quality in health care. The Department of Health's 1998 publication, *A First Class Service: Quality in the New NHS* [3], fails to define what is meant by quality!

Perhaps a better way to approach what we mean by quality is to reserve its use for those products and services that show excellence as perceived by the customer. There is no implied pecking order with excellence. There is no mountain of superiority. It is replaced by a broad spectrum of products and services which exhibit excellence in their numerous and diverse ways. Each product or service is judged by a customer on its own merits. Of course, different people have differing views as to what constitutes excellence in a product or service, and so the author's definition of quality is:

> Quality is excellence as perceived by a customer or a stakeholder. [4]

The above definition is also applicable to hospitals by replacing 'customer' by 'patient'. Thus, in hospital situations the definition becomes:

> Quality is excellence as perceived by a patient or a stakeholder.

Moreover, this definition puts the patient at the focus of all hospital work.

Another point to bear in mind in connection with 'quality' is that its meaning changes. Our views of what constitutes excellence in products or excellence in services, including excellence in hospital care, have been enhanced as a result of advances in modern science and technology. Quality, excellence as perceived by today's customers and stakeholders, is certainly different from what was perceived as quality in the past, even the recent past.

Quality assurance

Hospital staff members also need to understand the significance of quality assurance.

The author has defined 'quality assurance' as follows:

> Quality assurance is a pledge to a customer that the quality (as seen, demonstrated,

> defined, agreed and accepted) will be maintained for a particular product or a particular service.

When people buy shirts from a high street retailer, they know that they are buying a shirt of a grade decided by the retailer. The retailer will choose the materials or approve the materials, design the shirt, or approve the design. More importantly, if you were to go on a shopping spree and were to buy several shirts of the same design, you would expect them to be not merely similar, but to be exactly the same. That is what is meant by quality assurance. It is clear that 'quality assurance', unlike 'quality', is an objective term.

Consider again the author's definition for quality assurance when it is applied to a hospital:

> Quality assurance is a pledge to a *patient,* that the quality (as seen, demonstrated, defined, agreed and accepted) will be maintained for a particular patient or a particular service.

First, consider the product of a hospital. The product of a hospital as defined above is the 'improved quality of life of the patient' that leaves a hospital after diagnosis and treatment. Whatever the diagnosis and whatever the treatment, the patient outcomes will vary, even when patients have been diagnosed with the same problem. Of course, very many patients are able to lead a better quality of life after their diagnosis and treatment; others will not do so. With patients there will be a range of outcomes, however good the clinicians and whatever medical science and technology is available. It is for this reason that the author believes that the term quality assurance should not to be used when referring to patients in a hospital.

The term quality assurance can be applied to some of the clinical services and other services provided in a hospital. Thus, clinical services, such as recording an ECG, taking an X-ray, carrying out a CT scan, and taking an angiogram could all be quality assured if they are carried out by competent staff in accordance with procedures. Similarly, some non-clinical services, e.g. the hospital laundry and the sterilization of instruments, might be considered to be quality assured if the work is carried out as specified and suitable controls are in place to ensure that requirements are being met. In all such quality assured services the processes will have been followed precisely, and confidence in the outcomes is very high.

It is evident that the term quality assurance should be used with care in all hospital work.

Customers, patients and stakeholders

The customers of NHS hospital acute trusts are the patients. Since April 2003, the primary care trusts (PCTs) provide about 75% of the funds for acute hospitals. They obtain their funding from government. The 28 strategic health authorities also provide some funding for acute hospitals for specific purposes, e.g. training. The government obtains its funds from the British taxpayer. All these fund providers are the stakeholders of the NHS. The needs of all these stakeholders have to be addressed along with the needs of patients.

The way forward

If clinicians and other staff work closely with top management within a framework of a quality management system based on ISO 9001, and if clinical audit comes into its own in an atmosphere of openness, integrity and responsibility (the underlying tenets of clinical governance), then there is no reason why the NHS cannot again become the envy of the world. This book is intended to give guidance to all those working in the NHS who aspire to contribute to such an achievement as a provider of quality patient care.

Similar arguments will apply to the new government funded treatment centres in the UK that are run by private companies. Some may already have achieved certification to the standard, as is already the case with many private hospitals in the UK and elsewhere.

Chapter 2: Hospital documentation

Hospital documentation is a generic term that includes all the documents, records and data used in a hospital. Personal experience indicates that there is some confusion over the names given to different documents in a hospital. In this chapter an attempt is made to clarify this matter. Experience also shows that some of the contents in one document may be repeated in several documents. The introduction of ISO 9001 into a hospital should provide an opportunity for some rationalization of the existing documentation.

Some hospitals are in the process of computerizing all their documentation. This is to be encouraged, but the arguments below will still stand whether or not this is the case.

Hospital codes

Hospital codes are commonly used to differentiate between one hospital and another. It is common practice to derive these from the name of the hospital, for example, the Royal Berkshire Hospital might use a code such as RBH.

Policy documents

A policy document in a hospital is one issued by or on behalf of top management. A policy document applies throughout the hospital to all staff whatever their position in the hospital.

A few examples of policy documents are:

- quality policy;
- quality objectives;
- the organization chart;
- confidentiality within the hospital;
- communications with the media;
- release of medical records;
- sickness and absence;

maternity leave;

standards of dress;

disciplinary issues;

appeals;

grievances.

It is recommended that policy documents are given the prefix PL and a number, such as 101 upwards, for any new documents created in connection with the new quality management system.

Three very important policy documents are referred to in Chapter 5:

Quality policy, PL 101 (see page 35)

Quality objectives, PL 102 (see page 36)

The organization chart, PL 103 (see figure 5.1)

When any existing policy documents are revised, they should be renumbered if a new numbering system has been introduced as a result of preparation for ISO 9001 certification. Since policies are documents for the entire hospital there is no need to identify a department.

Departmental codes

Departmental codes are often used throughout hospitals in order to link a particular document with a specific department. Suggested codes are listed at the end of this chapter.

Thus, the Cardiology Department in the Sheffield Hallamshire Hospital might be indicated by: SHH CARD.

Processes and process diagrams

All hospitals will use processes and some will already have process diagrams in place, which are indicated by PD (see Chapter 3). Thus, an endocrinology process diagram in Glasgow Western Infirmary might be identified by: GWI ENDO PD 102 issue 2. (Glasgow Western Infirmary, Endocrinology Department, process diagram, number 102 and issue 2).

Procedures

A procedure explains how things are to be done. They give sufficient detail for the staff for whom they are written to do things as required. They are often supplementary to process diagrams and give details that cannot be stated on process diagrams.

Procedures can be identified by PC, and uniquely identified. For example, by RGH ENT PC 111, issue 3 (RGH for Rotherham General Hospital, a procedure in the Ears, Nose and Throat department, number 111 and issue 3).

See Appendix 1 for an example of the mandatory procedures required by ISO 9001.

Protocols

Protocols are similar to procedure documents with the important difference that they are consensual documents for clinicians and nursing staff clearly stating how patients are to be treated. They are usually written by hospital consultants who have the knowledge and experience to decide how patients are to be treated in their own departments. In preparing such protocols, consultants will be aware of evidence-based medicine and any other guidelines issued by the Department of Health and professional bodies.

Protocols can be indicated by PT and uniquely identified. For example, BH PT A&E 121, issue 1 (BH for Barnet Hospital, a protocol in the Accident & Emergency Department, number 121, issue 1).

Work instructions

Work instructions give step-by-step instructions on how a specific task must be performed. No deviations are allowed without the specific authority of a senior member of staff, who thereby accepts full responsibility for any such deviations.

Work instructions can be indicated by WI and uniquely identified. For example, GRI WI CD 151, issue 2 (GRI for Glasgow Royal Infirmary, a work instruction in the Cardiology department, number 151, issue 2)

Forms

Hospitals use many forms: hospital forms and departmental forms. The classification and numbering of forms will probably enable some rationalization to take place.

Forms can be indicated by FM and uniquely identified. For example, SHH FM HR 201, issue 1 (SHH for Sheffield Hallamshire Hospital, form used in the Human Resources department, number 201, issue 1).

External forms

If external forms are used or have to be completed by a hospital, each will have a unique number. There is no point in the hospital giving them additional numbers. External forms should simply be listed in whatever ways that the hospital decides are convenient. Groups of numbers might be allocated for different kinds of form.

External forms can be indicated by EFM and uniquely identified by a number only. For example, Department of Health EFM 001, 002, etc. or Professional Bodies EFM 101, 102, etc.

External documents

External documents can be listed in a similar way to external forms. They can be indicated by ED and uniquely indicated by a number only. For example, Department of Health ED 001, 002, etc. or Professional bodies ED 101, 102, etc.

Hospital records

Hospital records provide evidence about what has happened to patients whilst they are in a hospital or visiting a hospital for diagnosis or treatment. These include:

- patient case notes;
- X-rays;
- ultrasound scans;
- CT scans;
- ECGs.

All such records need to be suitably annotated, uniquely identified and preserved for future reference. The time that records must be kept are specified by law.

Quality management system documentation

When a hospital decides to seek certification to ISO 9001, additional documentation and records need to be created in order to control the quality management system. These are explained in Chapter 4 and are intended to be few in number. They are considered to be important for the quality management system and should enable management, clinicians and other staff to work closely together for the benefit of patients.

Some suggested hospital department codes

Accident and emergency	A&E
Anaesthesiology	ANAES
Cardiology	CD
Cardiothoracic surgery	CTS
Catering	CT
Dentistry	DT
Dermatology	DM
Dietary	DIE
Endocrinology	ED
Engineering	EG
Ears, nose and throat	ENT
Family medicine	FM
Finance	FN
Gastroenterology	GS
Housekeeping and laundry	H&L
Human resources	HR

Information technology	IT
Insurance	ID
Internal medicine	IM
Internal medicine and pulmonology	IM & PL
Interventional cardiology	IN CD
Medical physics	MP
Marketing	MK
Medical oncology	MO
Medical records	MR
Nephrology	NP
Neurology	NR
Nursing	NS
Obstetrics and gynaecology	OB & GN
Pharmacy	PH
Quality management system	QMS

Chapter 3: Process diagrams

Major processes and process diagrams

A process is simply a series of activities that are carefully planned and executed to achieve the desired objectives.

Any process is initiated through some form of input and the activities that follow will result in some form of output. In its simplest form, a process will consist of an input, one activity that adds value to the input, and a resulting output (as shown in Figure 3.1). In practice, many processes consist of a series of activities, each activity leading on directly to the next activity, each of which adds further value, ultimately resulting in the required output. Such a series of carefully planned activities constitute a more typical process (see Figure 3.2).

All organizations have at least one process: that is why an organization exists. This process is sometimes referred to as the major or primary process of an organization, as a core process, or as a first-level process.

In the case of large and complex organizations, it is usually extremely helpful to be able to establish the overall major process of the organization and the major process (or processes) in each department. This means that the departmental processes can be examined against the overall major process. In fact most organizations are likely to have more than one major process. A manufacturer might have a number of different product lines, each being controlled through a major process, whereas another organization might provide more than one service, each likewise being controlled by a major process.

All processes can be depicted in process diagrams, a number of which are shown at the end of this chapter (PD 101 to PD 107). Process diagrams are relatively easy to understand. They encourage all staff to focus on the output. Hopefully, the output for each major process will meet the needs and expectations of customers.

Lower-level processes

It is not always possible to show all the relevant information concerning a major process in one process diagram. It is for this reason that lower-level process diagrams are used. In other words, a major process diagram might be supported by lower-level diagrams usually referred to as second-level and third-level process diagrams. They can also be supported by notes attached to different stages in any of the processes.

Hospital process diagrams

Possible patient processes leading to diagnosis and treatment in hospitals

Process diagrams can, of course, be used to advantage in hospitals. Process diagram PD 101 shows one such example (see page 19). This process diagram gives an overview of the possible patient processes that a patient might take from the time of arrival at a hospital to the time that a patient leaves hospital. In a well-organized hospital, patient experiences will have been rationally planned so that the process of diagnosis and treatment will have proceeded in a logical and efficient manner. The result will have been the optimum use of the hospital's resources (doctors, nurses, support staff, equipment and facilities) with everyone acting in the best interest of patients. The ultimate goal is that the diagnosis and treatment will lead to patients having an improved quality of life as a result of attending hospital.

As some hospitals deal with hundreds of new patients each day, and also have to cope with a large number of in-patients who need some form of diagnosis, treatment and care, it is very important that all processes are well organized.

Every department in a hospital should have its own process diagram. This should show the logical steps that a patient undergoes prior to attending a department and after reaching the department. The mere preparation of a process diagram may result in improvements to the processes undertaken in the department. All staff should have access to the process diagram, which indicates in diagrammatic form what happens to patients as they progress, stage by stage through a department. In cases in which different departments are interdependent, a combined study of one or more interrelated process diagrams sometimes results in changes to the diagrams for the benefit of both staff and patients.

A major process in a hospital radiology department (first- and second-level)

Process diagram PD 102 shows 'A major process in a hospital radiology department' from the time that a patient arrives to the time of discharge. Note that in this case, PD 102 has one rectangle that has a black shadow on two sides. This indicates that one can proceed to the second-level process. Mistakes in this second-level process can cause problems and have a significant effect on the overall efficiency of the department. Indeed, every second-level process is there to ensure that the operational efficiency of the department is maximized at all times.

The major process in a hospital ECG department (first-level only)

The major process in an ECG department, PD 103, is similar to a major process in a radiology department.

The major process in the steam sterilization department of a dental hospital (first-level only)

The first level of process diagram PD 104 shows 'The steam sterilization of instruments in a dental hospital'. The flow diagram shows the routine process that instruments follow from the time that they leave the operating theatre to the time they are returned a few hours later, fully wrapped and sterilized and ready for reuse. The 'fast-steam' sterilization process shows how, in an emergency, instruments are sterilized without being wrapped and are returned to the operating theatre within minutes rather than by taking the standard route.

The process diagram also emphasizes the importance of sterilization records. It shows the importance of the essential work that is necessary to ensure that sterilization is achieved as planned.

The major process of out-patient appointments, diagnosis and/or treatment (first-level only)

Process diagram PD 105 shows how a modern yet simple out-patients' appointments system should function and provide data for management and any other interested parties.

Patient complaints (first-level only, but with notes attached to some stages)

Process diagram PD 106 shows how all patient complaints should be addressed in a systematic manner based on the latest document from the Department of Health, *NHS Complaints Reform: Making Things Right* [5].

Collection of information and data on patients in hospitals (first-level only)

Process diagram PD 107 shows a patient experience from referral to a hospital through to the time of discharge after surgery. Different hospitals might follow different procedures but whatever flow diagram is derived after consultation with all parties in a given hospital, all diagrams should enable some useful information and data to be collected on patients.

There are two key aspects to the collection of information and data: the first concerns diagnosis and treatment and the second concerns timing. Collecting information on timing is a relatively new development, which importantly puts the patient as the focus of attention in the NHS.

Information and data on patients can be collected at numerous stages in the process diagram PD 107 and also other stages that are not shown in the process diagram. Increasingly, all information from tests, X-rays, scans and other procedures and associated data will be stored on a hospital computer system. All processes related to the collection, collation and analysis of data will continue to improve as computer technology and its application to patient diagnosis and treatment continue to progress.

The same application of computer technology on timing can be used effectively with little effort. The most important time period for the patient is that between the GP requesting a hospital appointment and the patient being admitted for treatment (i.e. the time between stages 1 to 11). The most important time period is not the time between a diagnosis and the patient being admitted to hospital for treatment. If the time of receipt of a letter for an appointment were entered into a computer (stage 1) and the date that a hospital appointment given was likewise entered into the computer system (stage 2), then the time between the two would be calculated and stored for continuing collation and analysis. Top management could then observe from time to time what was happening in a given department.

A report on one north London hospital issued by the Commission for Health Improvement (CHI) [6] shows that there was no such control in that particular hospital, where requests for ultrasound investigation were allowed to build without being addressed. If there had been proper control in that department, top management would have been able to download such data at regular intervals and take appropriate action as and when necessary without waiting for the findings of the CHI. In this case top management had not established a suitable reporting line and therefore the backlog of patients waiting for treatment had reached 2,700 before top management became aware of the problem.

Collection, collation and analysis of time-data on patients based on patient flow diagrams can be made readily available to top management.

Advantages of process diagrams

The mere preparation of process diagrams can help hospitals to rationalize their major processes with the minimum amount of textual documentation. Second-level diagrams enable more information to be available, or to be drawn upon, as and when required without making the first-level diagram too complicated. This argument can be extended 'downwards' to yet further levels that contain important information that may not be relevant to many of the people working in accordance with higher level process diagrams.

Once the processes have been set up, implemented and the different levels integrated (and perhaps with those of other departments), there is little doubt that opportunities will arise for continual improvements to be made in the functioning of a department, and thereby, in the functioning of a hospital. Furthermore, flow diagrams encourage and help all members of staff to collect relevant information and data on different aspects of the departmental workings. This too helps the department to become more efficient and moreover enables top management to monitor where problems are arising in the department.

None of this is bureaucratic. Flow diagrams and collection of information and data of the right kind, particularly using computers, provide a simple means of obtaining facts and findings so that top management can manage effectively in the interests of everyone, but especially of the patients.

Collection and analysis of such data is also a requirement of ISO 9001 to enable top management to be in control and to provide opportunities to continually improve the effectiveness of its quality management system (see Chapter 8).

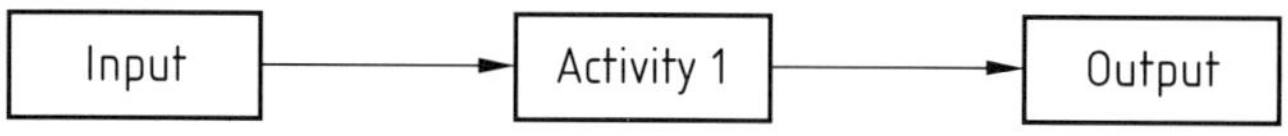

Figure 3.1 – A simple process

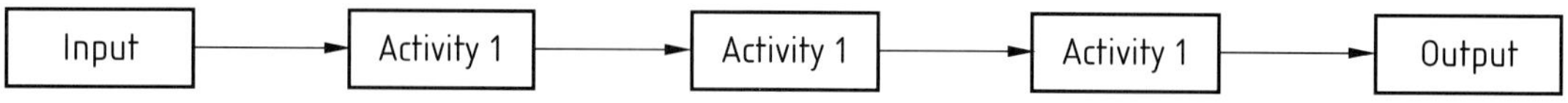

Figure 3.2 – A process showing consecutive activities

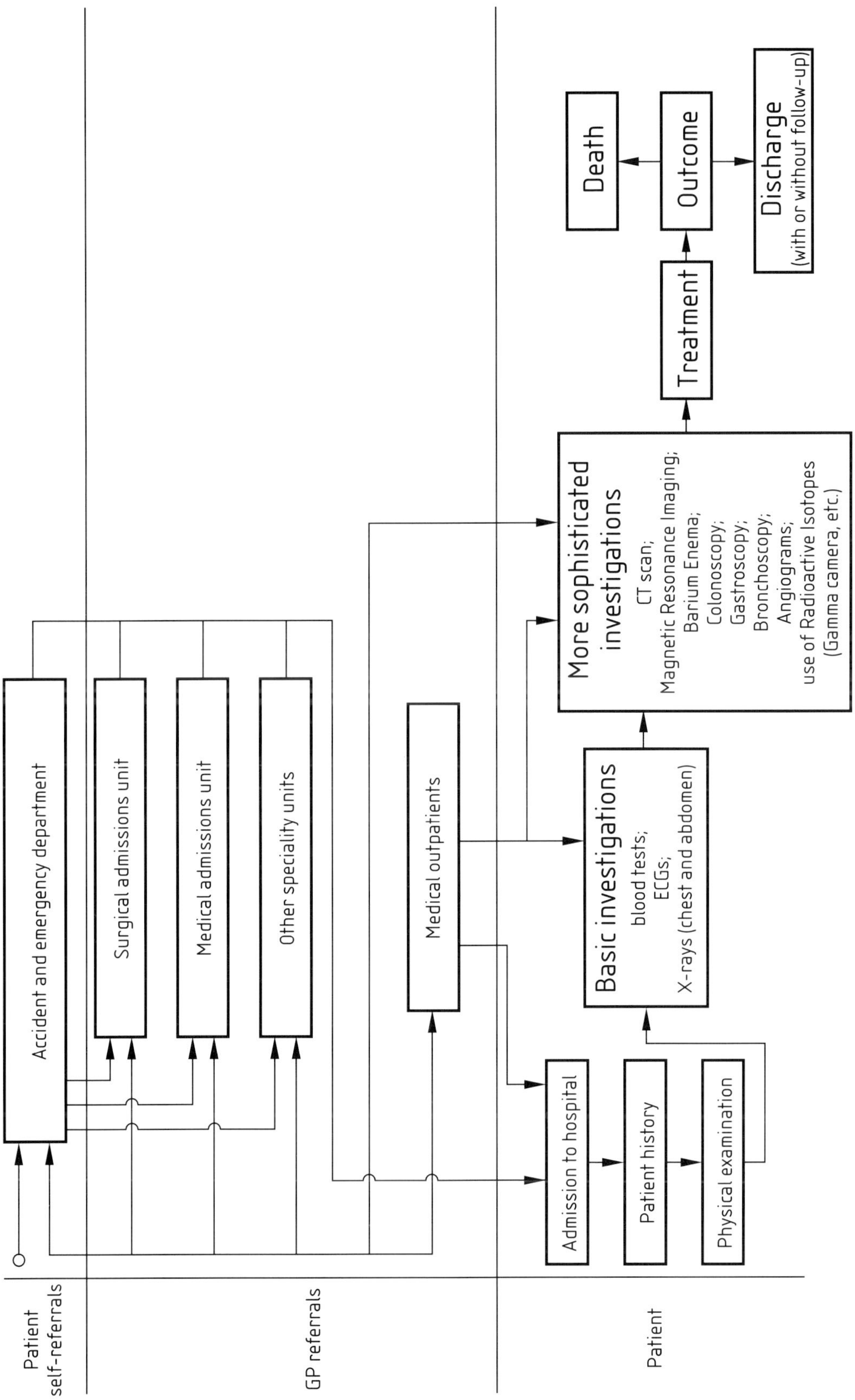

Figure 3.3 – Overview of a patient process in a hospital (PD 101)

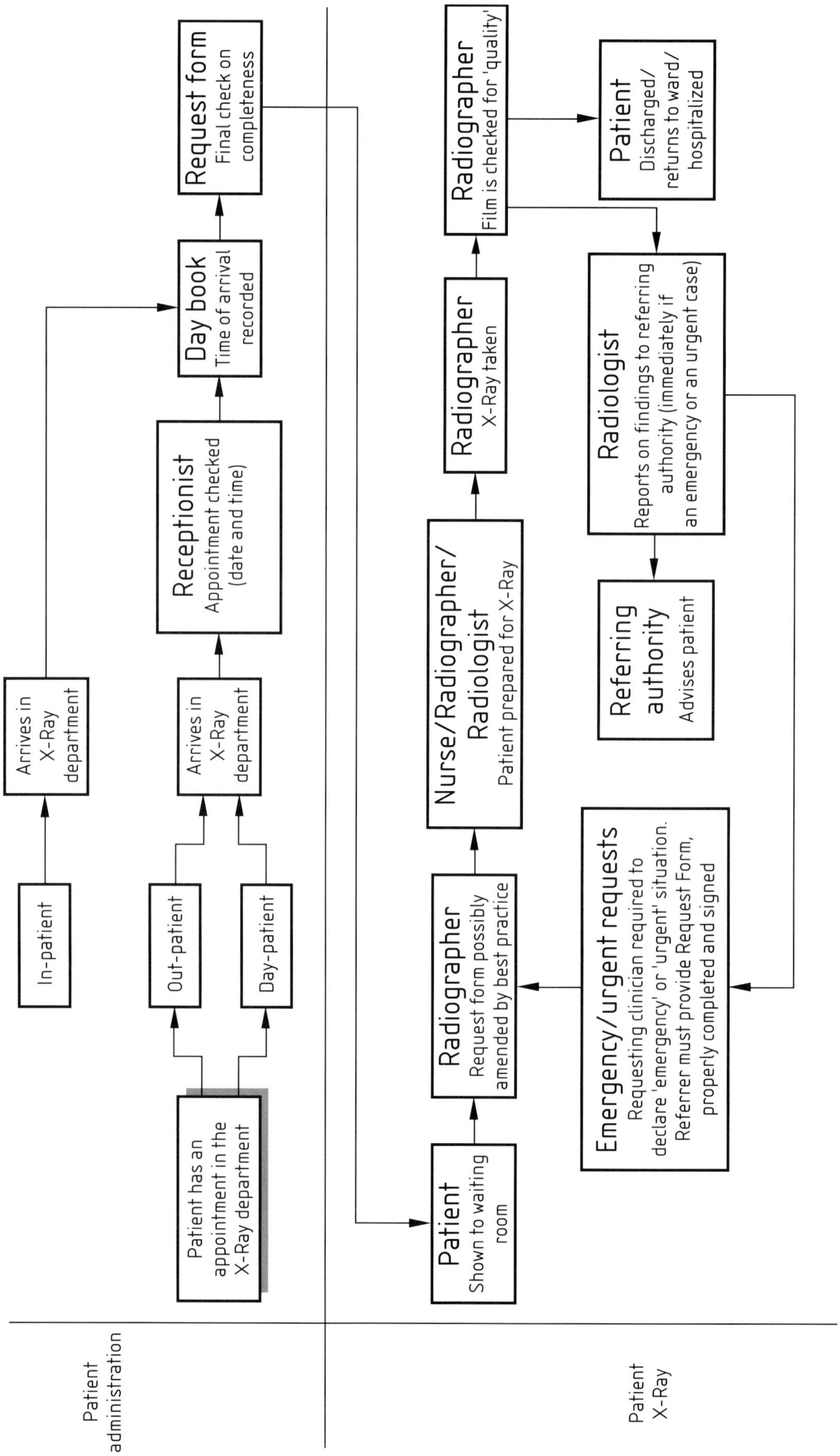

Figure 3.4a – A process in a hospital radiology department (PD 102)

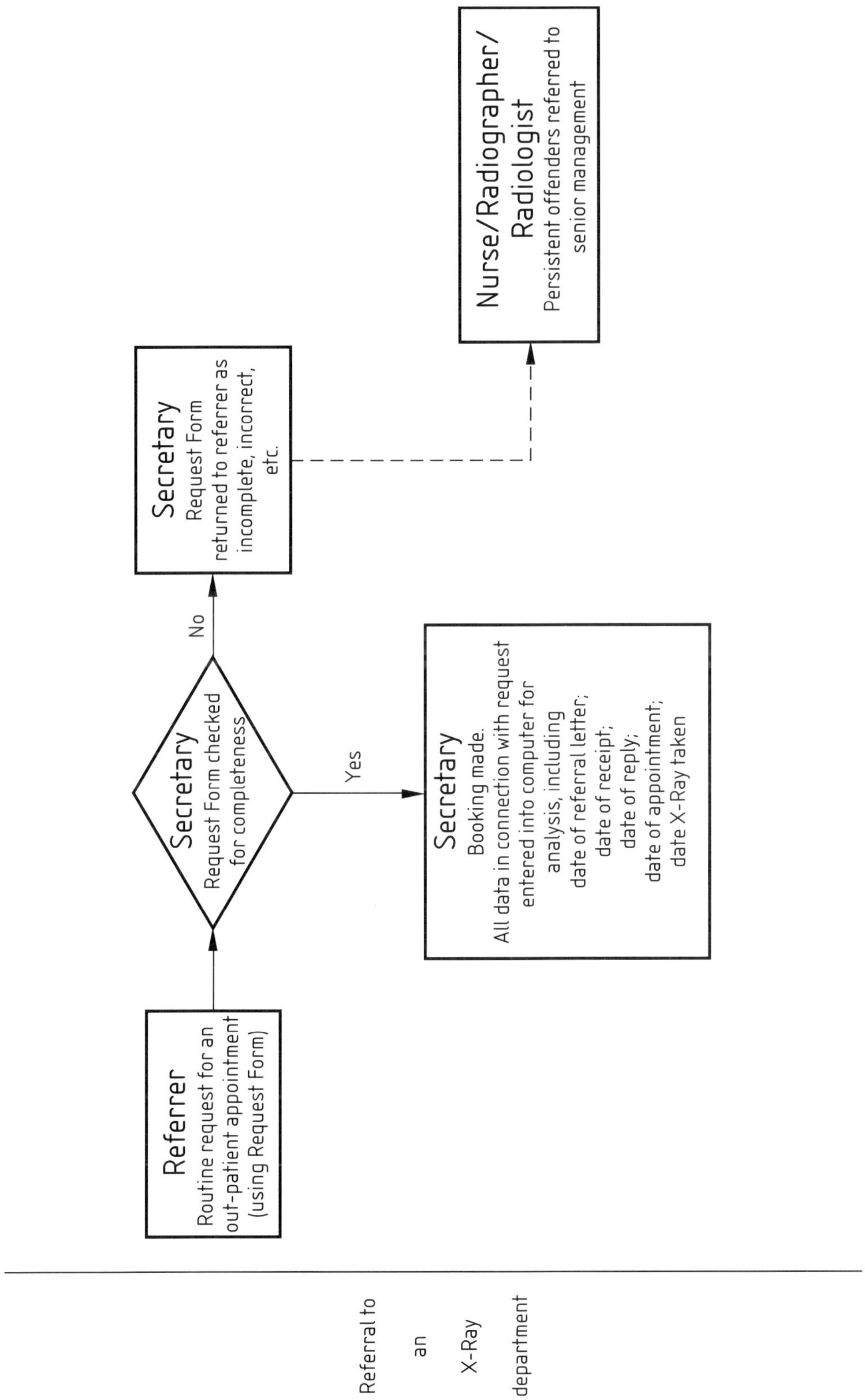

Figure 3.4b – A process for an X-Ray department (PD 102)

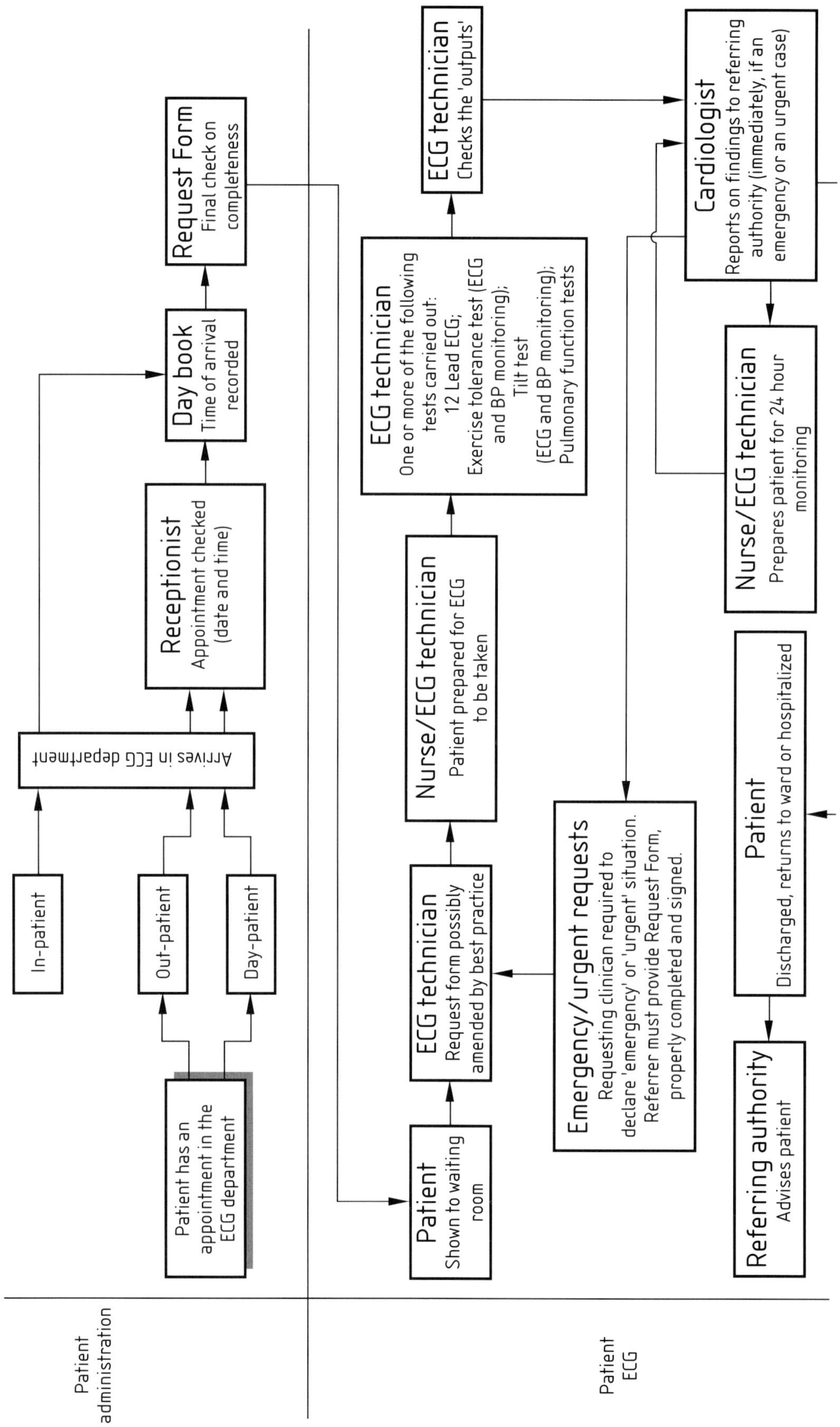

Figure 3.5 – A process in an ECG department (PD 103)

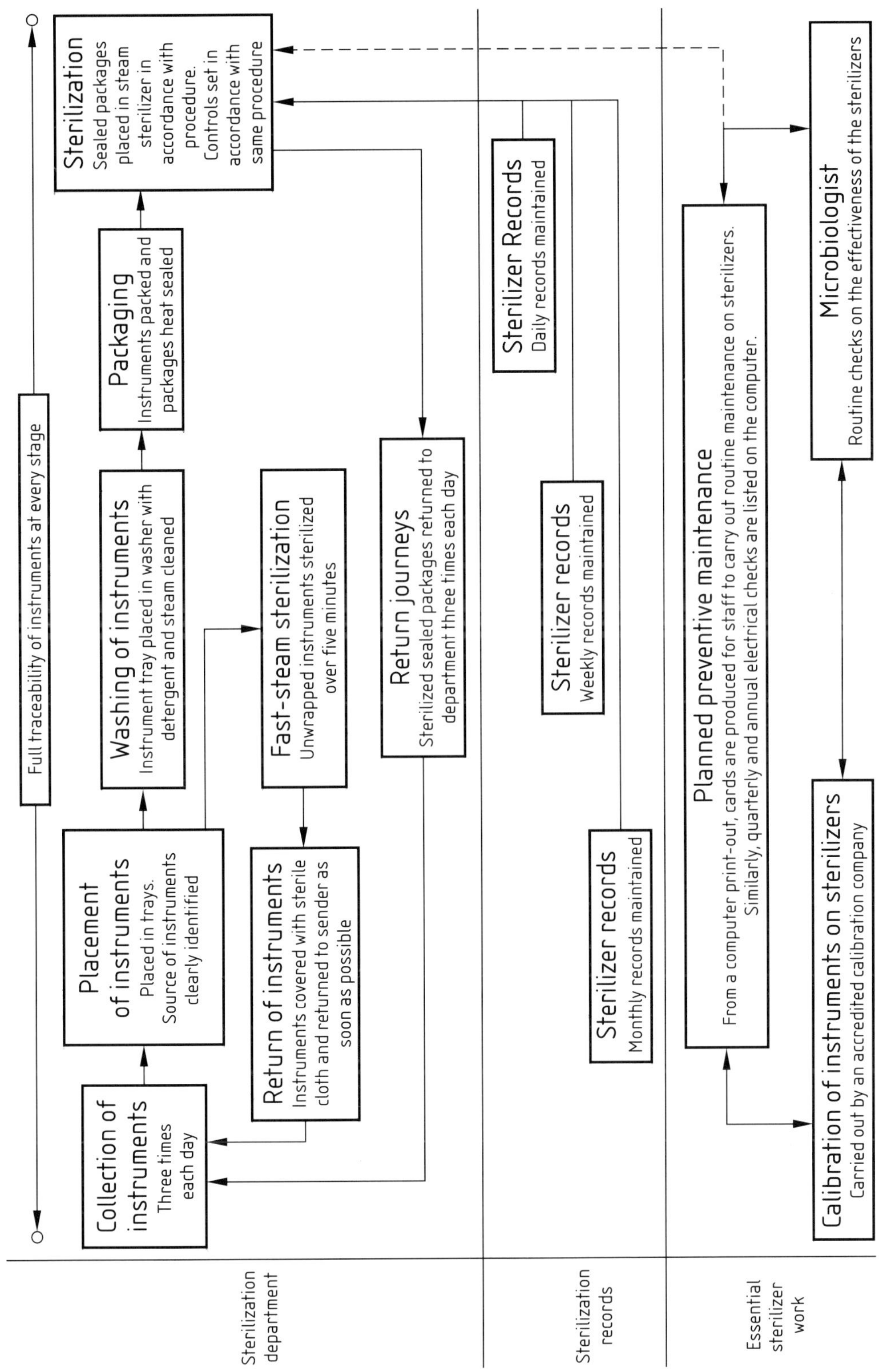

Figure 3.6 – Sterilization of instruments in a dental hospital (PD 104)

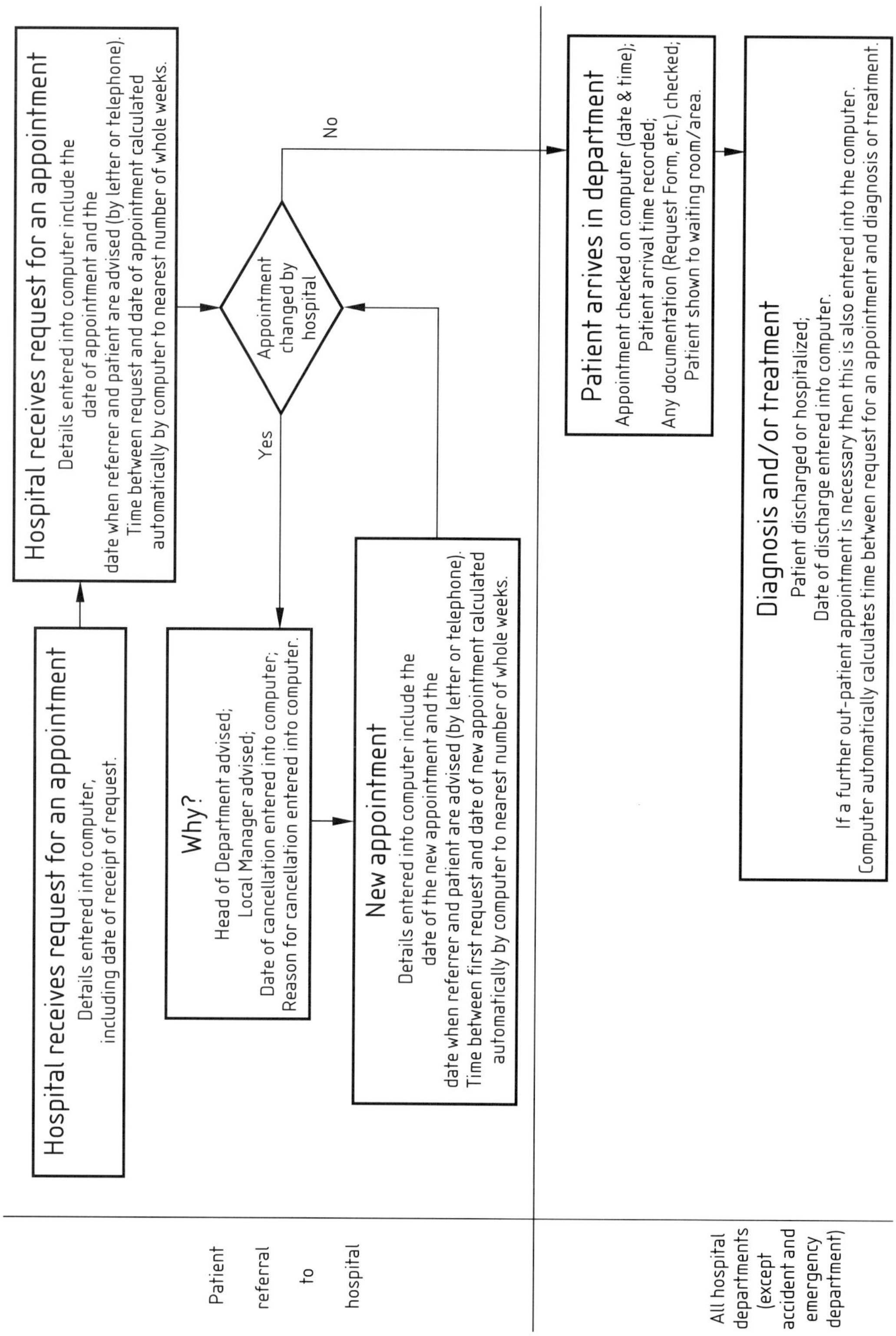

Figure 3.7 – A process for an out-patients' appointment system (PD 105)

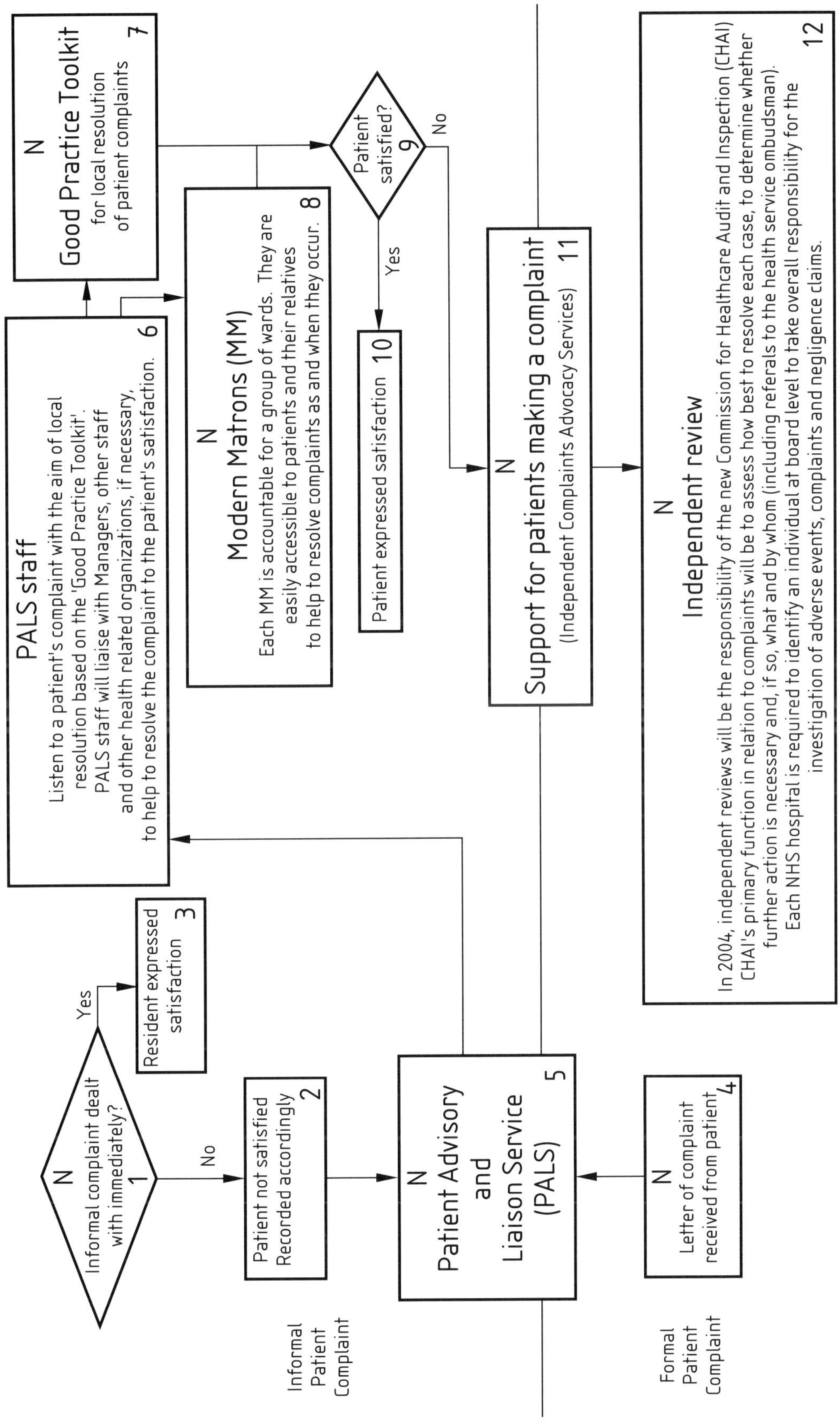

Figure 3.8 – A process for patient complaints (PD 106)

Notes attached to PD 106 on patient complaints

Stage 1: Informal complaints

Informal complaints might be verbal complaints on less serious matters that are nevertheless annoying to a patient. They can usually be addressed immediately by staff reponsible for the care of the patient by an apology followed immediately by appropriate action.

In the absence of an apology and especially if the complaint has not been dealt with in spite of repeated complaints, a small matter might become more serious. It should then be referred to the Patient Advisory and Liaison Service (PALS).

Stage 4: Formal complaints

In 2002, 140,000 patients made formal complaints that were dealt with through the NHS complaints procedure. Formal complaints tend to be more serious complaints, and they are submitted in writing to the hospital or to a member of staff of the hospital. In all such cases the letters must be referred to PALS without delay.

The Department of Health will promote the active management of complaints, and concerns of patients so that they are addressed as close as possible to when and where they arise and are responded to quickly, effectively and proportionately.

Stage 5: Patient Advisory and Liaison Service (PALS)

Every NHS trust and primary care trust in England is establishing its own Patient Advice and Liaison Service (PALS). The PALS remit is to address patients' complaints quickly and efficiently with minimum delays to the satisfaction of patients; and to use each and every complaint as a catalyst for possible changes and improvement.

Stage 7: Good practice toolkit

About 98% of patients' complaints are resolved locally.

Since the Spring of 2003, a 'Good Practice Toolkit' [5] has been available that draws on existing good practice. This document also provides a basis for consistent training and development. The toolkit promotes and encourages more open and flexible access to the complaints procedure. The maximum allowable time for local resolution of patient complaints is now 20 days.

The response to complaints must provide remedies that are closely tailored to the needs of patients, including explanations and apologies. Practical measures must be taken to put right what has gone wrong or is going wrong, as quickly and directly as possible.

Hospitals are expected to promote and facilitate the use of conciliation.

Stage 8: Indirect role of modern matrons

Modern matrons must demonstrate to nurses the high standards of care that NHS patients can expect. They must drive up standards of care and take a lead in providing advice on best professional practice and on patient services. They must also ensure that wards are clean, set and monitor standards and take action to ensure that any applicable cleaning specifications have been met.

Matrons must ensure that the nutritional needs of patients are met and ensure that patients get the right meals, at the right time and that they are able to eat their meals. The privacy and dignity of patients must be protected at all times.

Stage 11: Independent Complaints Advocacy Services (ICAS)

The government has to provide independent advocacy services to assist individuals making complaints against the NHS. ICAS will focus on helping individuals to pursue complaints about NHS services. The ICAS service will be available through: PALS, complaints managers at trust level, NHS Direct and through advertisements.

Stage 12: Independent review

In 2003-2004, over 90,122 people made a formal complaint [7]. Each year some thousands of patients requested an independent review.

A Department of Health evaluation report [5] on independent reviews came to the conclusion that:

> Independent Review is not perceived by complainants to be impartial. Improving this aspect of the current procedure is the single most commonly cited suggestion for reform.

It is for this reason that the government proposes to reform radically independent reviews of complaints by placing the responsibility for such independence with the new Commission for Healthcare Audit and Inspection (CHAI) (See Appendix 3).

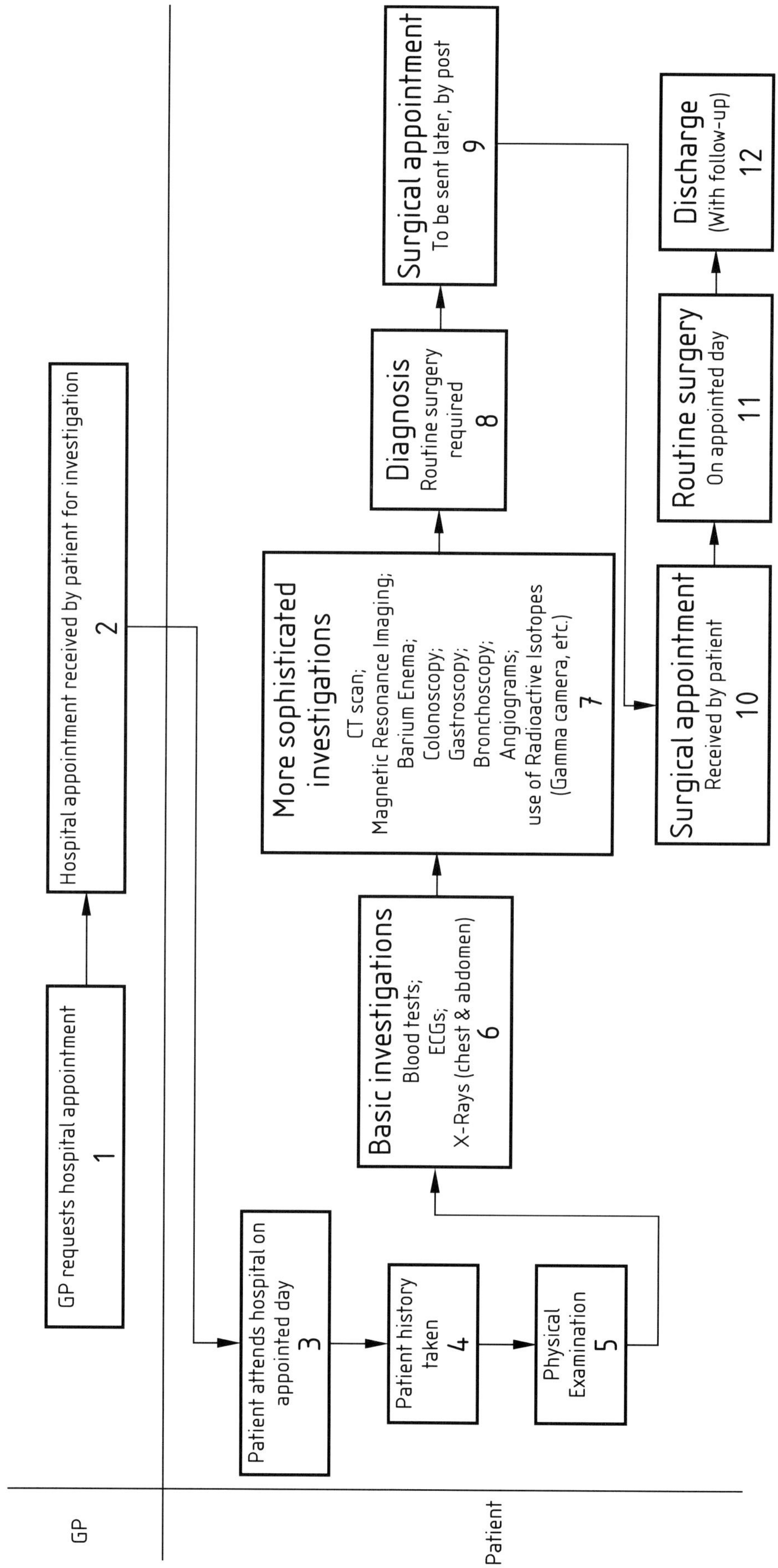

Figure 3.9 – Collection of information and data (PD 107)

Chapter 4:
Quality management system (clause 4)

General requirements (ISO 9001, clause 4.1)

Any hospital preparing for accredited certification to ISO 9001 must establish, document, implement and maintain a quality management system.

The documentation requirements of ISO 9001:2000 are less onerous than was required for the previous edition, ISO 9001:1994. Once the documentation has addressed certain basic requirements of the standard, the extent of the quality management system documentation can be decided by the hospital itself, depending on:

- the type of activities;
- the size of the hospital;
- the complexity and interaction of the processes;
- the competency of personnel.

Large complex hospitals with many employees will probably need more documentation than small hospitals. The hospital can decide whether the documentation is to be in hard copy throughout, or on a computer network or an intranet.

The standard focuses on processes. A hospital must clearly identify its major processes and any interactions with other major or supplementary processes, to ensure that they collectively result in quality patient care that achieves planned results and thereby satisfies the needs and expectations of patients. Management (see Chapter 5) must ensure that adequate resources are available and that relevant information and documentation are always available at appropriate stages during any of the processes. Above all, management has to ensure that all first-level processes and any interacting processes proceed in ways that achieve the planned results in the most efficient manner.

Hospitals already have many processes in place. Most were probably introduced informally and have been amended from time to time in the light of experience, new knowledge and new technology. Similarly, the satisfactory operation and control of such processes will have been brought to fruition in the light of such experience. Test criteria to be used at specific stages in a process may already be in place. Appropriate monitoring and measurements that have to be made continuously, or continually (i.e. from time to time), at different stages in a process may have been decided. Any data that are collected during such processes may already be collated and analysed from time to time. Any observations, monitoring and measurements might result in corrective actions being taken to put right what was going wrong or what has gone wrong. The standard ensures that processes, which might currently be informal arrangements, are formally introduced and controlled systematically.

Formalization of processes and controls is not to be regarded as a bureaucratic requirement. It enables all staff in all departments, but especially top management and senior medical staff, to understand how departments should function. Moreover, understanding how departments function provides opportunities for everyone within a department, and perhaps others outside a department, to promote continual improvement in the effectiveness of the new quality management system of the hospital. This is a prime requirement of the standard and it applies to all the activities that take place in the hospital.

Sometimes a hospital uses resources from outside to carry out tasks on its behalf. The standard refers to such actions as outsourcing.

A hospital might consider outsourcing an activity when:

- it is not a major or core process of the hospital;
- a hospital does not have the specialized knowledge and skills that are necessary to carry out certain processes. Whilst these could sometimes be acquired in-house it might be prohibitively expensive to do so.

Cleaning and security are examples of outsourcing. Such services were the forerunners of today's wide-ranging outsourcing services sector in which services are devolved to trusted external organizations.

If a hospital subcontracts, or outsources, any services that can affect patient care, directly or indirectly, then the hospital must maintain close control over such outsourcing. This means that it must be evident from the quality management system documentation of the hospital that outsourcing is tightly controlled.

Documentation requirements (ISO 9001, clause 4.2)

General (ISO 9001, clause 4.2.1)

Quality management system documentation can be conveniently divided into three main categories: the framework documentation, working documents and records (see Figure 4.1). The records are derived from both the framework documentation and from working documents. The framework documentation is the core documentation on which the quality management system is based. Working documents control all the activities in a hospital that are necessary to support the major processes. Management can claim to have a quality management system in place when it believes that all of its quality management system documentation has been implemented and that all employees are working in accordance with the planned arrangements.

The quality management system documentation must include a quality manual (see clause 4.2.2).

A quality policy statement is required (see page 35) and this must be a controlled document.

Quality objectives must be included in the quality management system documentation (see clause 5.4.1). Since these are likely to change from time to time, any changes can easily be made in a controlled manner by changing the issue number of the document that lists the quality objectives (see clause 4.2.3).

Only six mandatory documented procedures are required by the standard:

- control of documents (see clause 4.2.3);
- control of quality records (see clause 4.2.4);
- internal audit (see clause 8.2.2);
- control of nonconforming product (see clause 8.3);
- corrective action (see clause 8.5.2);
- preventive action (see clause 8.5.3).

Otherwise, a hospital is given complete freedom to decide what documentation is necessary to control the key aspects of the quality management system. It is also given complete freedom to decide what documentation is required to control the processes that ultimately result in planned patient care achieving a better quality of life for patients. Records are also required to be kept and maintained as explained below (see clause 4.2.4).

The framework documentation

The framework documentation is the core documentation required to establish and maintain the quality management system. In the experience of the author, the quality management system framework documentation detailed below appears to satisfy every conceivable situation.

All documents should be coded for classification purposes. In addition, all documents (with the exception of the quality manual) can be numbered, e.g. from 101 upwards, so that new quality management system documents can be readily identified. This does not, of course, mean that documents with numbers up to 100 are no longer relevant. Any such existing documents should continue to be used until the new quality management system has been established. Consideration can then be given to withdrawing any documents that have been superseded by the new quality management system or, if they are to be retained for inclusion in the new quality management system, they can continue to be used with any existing reference letters and/or numbers. When such documents are modified they can also be recoded and renumbered to fit in with the new arrangements in the new quality management system.

Suggested codes are as follows:

Quality management system manual	QM (see clause 4.2.2)
Quality management system process diagrams	PD 101, PD 102, etc.
Quality management system procedures	PC 101, PC 102, etc.
Quality management system policies	PL 101, PL 102, etc.
Quality management system forms	FM 101, FM 102, etc.
Quality management system external documents	ED 101, ED 102, etc.
Quality management system external forms	EFM 101, EFM 102, etc.

Note that external documents and external forms will normally already have a unique identification number. However, they can also be coded as above for control purposes.

Working documents

There is another important aspect to any quality management system, namely, working documents (see Figure 4.1). These are documents that a hospital considers necessary for planning, operation and control of all its processes. They will include patient case notes, X-rays, and scans amongst others. In addition, working documents might include protocols, procedures, policies, work instructions, forms, external documents and external forms. Hospitals will not necessarily have all the above categories of documentation. For instance, some organizations may decide that few work instructions are necessary. On the other hand, management and/or clinicians may decide that some other additional form of documentation is required in order to achieve the planned results or perhaps to prevent, or minimize, the likelihood of an untoward event happening again (see clause 8.2.3).

All hospitals are likely to have some external documents (other than the standard itself) issued from outside sources such as government departments and professional bodies. In the UK these will include documents such as those issued by the National Institute for Clinical Excellence (NICE) and the National Service Frameworks (NSF) (see Appendix 3).

Working documents will include any external forms imposed on the hospital for completion by, for example, the Department of Health.

Working documents are also used to control suppliers and subcontractors, but there will be no need for additional controls when a government department undertakes bulk purchases on behalf of hospitals.

Quality Manual (ISO 9001, clause 4.2.2)

A hospital must establish and maintain a quality management system manual. The quality manual must address the five requirement clauses of the standard.

These are:

- clause 4: quality management system;
- clause 5: management responsibility;
- clause 6: resource management;
- clause 7: product realization;
- clause 8: measurement, analysis and improvement.

Management can decide on the format of the quality manual.

A quality policy statement is required. This need not be included in the manual, although it often is. It is usually signed and dated by the chief executive. An example quality policy document is given on page 35. The standard requires it to be a controlled document.

The chief executive has to ensure that quality objectives are set at relevant functions and levels within the hospital. These quality objectives must be measurable and can also be formally issued as a policy document. Again, this ensures proper control and updating is facilitated. There must be a framework in place to ensure that quality objectives are systematically reviewed. Such reviews provide opportunities for top management to demonstrate its commitment to continual improvement in the effectiveness of its quality management system.

An organization chart is required. Organization charts frequently change and can best be controlled as a policy document (see Figure 5.1).

Scope and permissible exclusions

The quality manual must include the scope of the quality management system. All of the processes of diagnosis, treatment and care within the hospital will be reflected in the scope of the quality management system documentation and the scope of the ISO 9001 certificate.

If a hospital decides to extend its facilities, it can do so outside the current scope. For instance, if a hospital decides to establish an accident and emergency unit, it will provide appropriate facilities in terms of a building, wards, examination rooms and equipment. The process of establishing such a new unit would initially remain outside of the declared scope. Once the facilities have been provided, management would appoint professional staff to carry out the diagnostic and therapeutic work as one of its several major processes and the scope would have to be modified accordingly, by agreement with its certification body.

ISO 9001 is intended to be generic and applicable to all kinds of organizations, regardless of type and size, irrespective of the product being manufactured or the service being provided. However, it is accepted that all the requirements of the standard may not be applicable to all organizations. ISO 9001, 1.2, under scope, states that exclusion can be considered where the requirements of the standard cannot be applied, 'due to the nature of an organization and its product'. Such exclusions are, however, limited to the contents of clause 7 provided the exclusions do not affect the organization's ability, or responsibility, to provide a service that fulfils customer and applicable regulatory requirements. If requirements that are not permissible are excluded, or if exclusion of requirements are not adequately justified, then conformity to ISO 9001 cannot be claimed and an external auditor would not be able to recommend to their accredited certification body that a certificate be awarded. The exclusions must also be made clear in any other publicly available documents, such as certification documents or marketing documentation, to avoid misleading third parties such as patients, customers and stakeholders.

Justifiable exclusions in a hospital

The design and development clause (ISO 9001, 7.3) simply cannot be addressed for a hospital. A separate chapter (see Chapter 9) explains why this clause cannot be addressed.

Procedures

A procedure is merely the prescribed way in which an activity is carried out. Procedures can be in any form and format. Six procedures are mandatory, but management will almost certainly decide that other procedures are required in order to control its processes satisfactorily. All procedures can be included in the quality manual, but it is common practice to keep them separate. However, appropriate cross-references must be made to procedures in the text of the manual. It is also common practice to list all the procedures in an appendix to the manual.

Interaction between processes

The quality manual will contain many processes and from these it is possible, with the supporting documentation, to understand the interaction of all processes in the quality management system. Some process diagrams refer to other process diagrams, others may have access to lower-level processes and some may have attached notes.

Control of documents (ISO 9001, clause 4.2.3)

All the documents associated with the quality management system are controlled. The proper control of documents is essential to ensure that only the approved latest documents and forms are in use, even though changes to the documentation will inevitably be necessary from time to time. The management representative is usually made responsible for control of documents that form part of the quality management system of the organization. The mandatory procedure PC 101 explains how this is done.

Control of records (ISO 9001, clause 4.2.4)

Records are different from the other two groups of documentation. Records arise from the many activities that occur in a hospital and they help provide objective evidence about what has happened. ISO 9001 requires specific records defined in the standard to be kept and maintained for defined periods of time. They are referred to as records in this document. A hospital will have to add other records to the list, such as patient records, many of which have to be kept and maintained because of statutory or regulatory requirements. The mandatory procedure PC 102 explains how records are controlled.

The hospital must decide on the minimum retention times for the different kinds of records. In certain cases the times are specified by external organizations. There must be explicit arrangements for disposition of records after the minimum retention times have been reached.

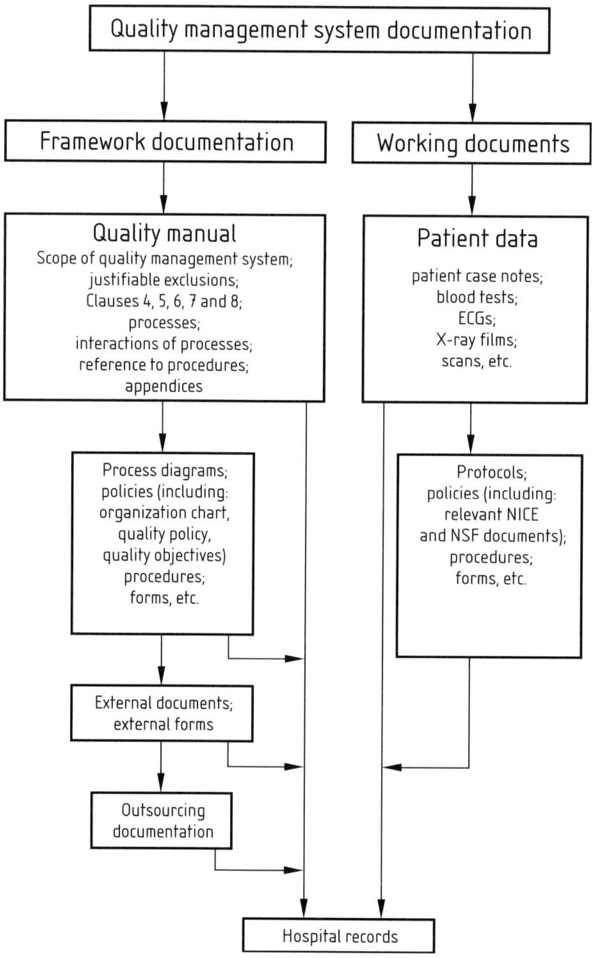

Figure 4.1 Quality management system documentation

Quality Policy

The hospital is a 1,000 bedded NHS hospital offering quality patient care in a caring and friendly environment. The hospital provides a complete range of in-patient and out-patient care in general medicine and surgery, together with many speciality units that are fully equipped with state of the art technology. It extols its centres of excellence such as its 30 bed Intensive Care Unit; an Accident and Emergency Unit in which waiting times are kept to an absolute minimum; an Obstetrics and Gynaecology Unit and a Cardiology Department, all of which work towards being second to none in the UK.

Staffing of the hospital has proved to be little of a problem since the hospital's standing in healthcare is excellent. Even so, top management, medical staff, nursing staff and other professional staff allied to healthcare are all committed to further improvement of the level of healthcare provided by the hospital.

All staff of the hospital are committed to excellence based on the International Quality Management System Standard, ISO 9001:2000.

The hospital management is committed to providing leadership for continual improvement in the effectiveness of its quality management system. Measurable quality objectives are in place, which are reviewed on a regular basis in a systematic manner at management review meetings. These include overall quality objectives for the hospital and specific objectives for each department,

The hospital strives at all times to achieve complete patient satisfaction. Patient satisfaction is monitored so that improvements can always be made when any shortcomings are identified.

All staff, including new employees, are made aware of the quality management system and are expected to implement, maintain and adhere to its requirements. Everyone is encouraged to suggest ways in which the quality management system can be improved.

The hospital management will review this quality policy statement at least annually, or earlier when considered to be appropriate.

Date: .... Signed: ....

Chief Executive of the Hospital

Quality Objectives

(Each NHS Hospital Trust must determine what its most important objectives are and which of these should be set for, say, the ensuing year. Those given below are merely suggestions.)

Hospital objectives

To reduce the number of formal patient complaints by 20% during the 12 months beginning November 2005.

To establish by January 2006 an independent review stage for complainants who remain dissatisfied by the response they have received from the attempts to resolve matters locally.

Departmental objectives

To ensure that all written requests for hospital appointments are given by letter within 14 days of receipt.

All changes to appointments will be recorded along with the reasons for those changes.

By 2006, nobody should have to wait more than four hours in the Accident and Emergency department from time of arrival to hospital admission/transfer elsewhere/discharge.

Waiting times for routine out-patient and in-patient treatment will be systematically recorded.

By 2006, maximum waiting time for routine out-patient appointment is to be three months.

By 2006, maximum waiting time for in-patient treatment is to be six months.

The hospital's management will review these quality objectives on a systematic basis at least annually, or earlier when considered to be appropriate.

Date: .... Signed: ....

Chief Executive of the Hospital

Chapter 5:
Management responsibility (clause 5)

Management commitment (ISO 9001, clause 5.1)

Each requirement in clause 5 of ISO 9001 begins: 'Top management shall'. In the case of the NHS hospitals in the UK this refers to the chief executives together with their senior colleagues. It is they who are ultimately responsible for directing and controlling a hospital.

The chief executives of hospitals are not able to absolve themselves from all responsibilities that arise from a quality management system based on ISO 9001. The new standard places explicit responsibilities on top management. This should mean that top management will be actively involved in the quality management system of the hospital. As a result, managers at lower-levels are much more likely to take a greater interest in it.

An external auditor will require objective evidence of the commitment of top management to the development, implementation and continuing improvement in the effectiveness of the quality management system based on ISO 9001:2000. Top management has to establish a quality policy (see clause 5.3); they have to ensure that quality objectives are set, measured and reviewed from time to time (see clause 5.4); they have to conduct management reviews (see clause 5.6); they have to ensure the availability of adequate resources (see Chapter 6); and they must ensure that all employees are made aware of the importance of striving at all times to improve the quality of the lives of all patients, while at the same time satisfying any statutory and regulatory requirements in connection with patient care in hospitals. (It is axiomatic that clinicians responsible for patient care will be aware of statutory and regulatory requirements.) Thus, if a hospital is seeking certification to the standard, top management can no longer absolve itself from all the activities associated with the standard, as some might argue was the case with the precursor of the current standard.

Customer focus (ISO 9001, clause 5.2)

Top management must be patient orientated. Patients tend to think increasingly that they will leave hospital with an improved quality of life, within any limitations imposed by the ever widening boundaries of modern medical science and technology. But patients have other expectations, for example they expect to experience common courtesies, cleanliness at all times and in all places in the hospital and good food, all of which are accepted as being part of life in our modern society. Fortunately, many of the changes that have been taking place in our hospitals over the last few years, irrespective of ISO 9001, have gradually been introduced for the benefit of patients, to the credit of top management and other staff.

The revised standard focuses on processes and this might simply mean formalizing patient processes that already exist. On the other hand, patient processes might never have been considered before. Development and improvement in patient processes have one aim, namely that of enhancing patient satisfaction (see clauses 7.1 and 8.2.1).

Top management has to decide how to monitor patient satisfaction: how to collect relevant information from patients and how to examine the information collected (see clause 8.2.1).

Quality policy (ISO 9001, clause 5.3)

Top management is responsible for the quality policy statement, which is a controlled document. An example quality policy statement is provided on page 35. The quality policy must be appropriate, i.e. relevant to the purpose of the hospital. It should contain commitments that are realistic and attainable.

The quality policy statement must include a commitment not only to satisfying the requirements of ISO 9001, but there must also be a commitment continually to improve the effectiveness of the quality management system of the hospital.

The quality policy statement must state that a framework exists for reviewing all measurable quality objectives in a systematic manner.

Top management has the responsibility for ensuring that all employees (including new employees) fully understand the quality policy statement. All managers should be encouraged to discuss the implications of the quality policy statement with the people for whom they are responsible.

Top management must look at the quality policy statement in a systematic way to review its continuing suitability. It is good practice to have the quality policy on the standard agenda of management reviews, as a reminder that it is to be reviewed at least once each year. This may be at the first review meeting in the year, or when the need arises because of changes within the hospital.

There is no requirement for the quality policy statement to be included in the quality manual. However, it is good practice for the quality policy statement to be made into a stand-alone policy document and displayed at strategic points within the hospital. It should be written on the hospital's headed paper, be signed by one or more members of top management and dated, thus signifying its importance and providing evidence to all employees and other interested parties that top management is committed to the quality management system of the hospital. The quality policy statement can be uniquely identified, e.g. PL 101, Issue 1.

Planning (ISO 9001, clause 5.4)

Quality objectives (ISO 9001, clause 5.4.1)

There is an explicit emphasis on quality objectives. Quality objectives [see clause 4.2.1(a)] must be established at relevant functions and levels within the hospital, including those needed for the patients [see clauses 5.4.1 and 7.1(a)]. Quality objectives must be measurable and consistent with the quality policy statement. There must also be a framework for reviewing quality objectives systematically as stated in an hospital's quality policy statement [see clause 5.3(c) and the example quality policy statement on page 35]. Such reviews provide opportunities for top management to demonstrate its commitment to continual improvement in the effectiveness of the quality management system.

Like the quality policy statement, it is good practice for the quality objectives statement to be made into a stand-alone document and displayed at strategic points within the hospital. If it is written on the hospital's headed paper, and signed and dated by one or more members of top management, then this should signify its importance. This statement will provide evidence to all employees and other interested parties that top management is committed to the quality management system of the hospital. The quality objectives can be uniquely identified, e.g. PL 102, Issue 1.

As top management is responsible for ensuring that quality objectives are set and measured, quality objectives should receive a new impetus and importance.

There are two opportunities to set quality objectives. The first opportunity is at the planning stages across the whole spectrum of a hospital's activities and departmental levels, including quality objectives that are relevant for satisfying the requirements for patients. The second opportunity is after implementation of the quality management system or, if this has already been implemented, after the introduction of any new processes. Feedback from these activities might identify the need for changes to be made to quality objectives or the introduction of additional quality objectives.

It is such feedback that provides an opportunity for continually improving the effectiveness of the quality management system. A failure to show continual improvement in the effectiveness of the quality management system, as determined by the measurements made in connection with the quality objectives set, would indicate the need for further investigations and perhaps for additional, or amended, quality objectives. An external auditor from a certification body would be able to make only an observation against such a failure, not a nonconformity, for there may be many reasons why a hospital has failed to meet certain quality objectives. (An auditor may at the same audit be satisfied by other objective evidence that the hospital is nevertheless continually striving to improve the effectiveness of its quality management system.)

Different hospitals pursuing different activities will choose different targets to focus on, depending on what is most important to the hospital.

Quality management system planning (ISO 9001, clause 5.4.2)

When planning the quality management system, top management must ensure that the general requirements of the quality management system are addressed (see clause 4.1) as well as any quality objectives such as those referred to in the commentary to clause 5.4.1.

Top management must ensure that the integrity of the quality management system is maintained when changes to it are planned and implemented.

Responsibility, authority and communication (ISO 9001, clause 5.5)

Responsibility and authority (ISO 9001, clause 5.5.1)

Top management must ensure that lines of responsibility and authority are defined and communicated within the hospital. This is essentially no different from the former standard except that it emphasizes the obvious, namely, the need to communicate the different responsibilities and authorities of personnel within the hospital.

One simple and effective method of doing this is for a hospital organization chart to be issued (see Figure 5.1). It is given an issue number that can be amended each time a change takes place. There is no need for names of staff to be included in the hospital chart, but within the framework of the specified hospital, the responsibilities and authorities of senior staff must be made known throughout the hospital. The hospital's organization chart can be uniquely identified, e.g. PL 103, Issue 1.

Management representative (ISO 9001, clause 5.5.2)

Top management must appoint a management representative from amongst it own staff. Other titles may be used for management representative, such as quality manager, quality director and quality coordinator. The hospital should use whatever it deems most appropriate.

The management representative has a number of defined responsibilities. First, the management representative has to ensure that the processes for the quality management system are established, implemented and maintained. The management representative has to report to top management on the performance of the quality management system and on any changes that should be made in order, for instance, to increase the operational efficiency of the hospital. The management representative has to ensure the promotion of awareness of patient requirements throughout the hospital. This latter requirement is a new explicit one.

A management representative might have other related responsibilities, such as liaison with external parties on the quality management system. In practice, a management representative plays a key role in the quality management system of a hospital. Typical responsibilities are:

- establishment, implementation and maintenance of the quality management system;
- reporting to top management on the performance of the quality management system and the need for changes for whatever reasons;
- promoting the awareness of patient requirements throughout the hospital; (The prime requirement is an improved quality of life for all patients. Secondary requirements include privacy, common courtesies, cleanliness, good food. Clinicians and other staff also have their parts to play in achieving these requirements.)
- arranging, in consultation with other people, the internal audit programme; arranging internal quality audits; arranging consequential corrective and preventive actions, if any;
- nonconformities: corrective actions and preventive actions;
- patient and stakeholder complaints; corrective and preventive actions;
- approval of suppliers and subcontractors;
- establishment and maintenance of supplier and subcontractor lists;
- control of calibrations of inspection, measuring and test equipment;

- collection and analysis of data for presentation to the management review meetings;
- the arrangement of the management review meetings;
- preparation and maintenance of records, archiving of records and data;
- liaison with certification bodies and other external hospitals and people on all matters relating to the quality management system.

This list of responsibilities of the management representative is not intended to be exhaustive.

Internal communication (ISO 9001, clause 5.5.3)

Top management must ensure that appropriate communication processes are established within the hospital and that the lines of communication between different people at different levels in the hospital are established and clearly understood within the hospital.

Top management can choose whatever other methods are considered to be most effective in establishing first-class communications with its staff. These might include:

1. meetings on the hospital's vision for the future;
2. meetings focusing on the immediate prospects for the future;
3. general meetings held on a regular basis with all staff;
4. departmental meetings;
5. meetings that focus on feedback from staff;
6. meetings on the suggestion scheme awards;
7. merit recognition meetings;
8. use of notice boards for imparting important information;
9. in-house journals or magazines.

Regular meetings might be held exclusively in connection with ISO 9001, at which any aspect of the quality management system can be discussed.

Specifically, feedback to top management regarding the effectiveness of the quality management system will be encouraged. This might be achieved through regular meetings, individual representations, or written submissions. Top management will stress to all employees the importance of such feedback.

Management review (ISO 9001, clause 5.6)

General (ISO 9001, clause 5.6.1)

Top management must review the hospital's quality management system at planned intervals to ensure its continuing suitability, adequacy and effectiveness. The review must include assessing opportunities for improvement and the need for changes to the quality management system, including changes to the quality policy and quality objectives.

There is no requirement regarding the frequency of management reviews. The hospital is completely free to decide the planned interval between such meetings. However, it is evident that meetings that are held only annually cannot be of any real value to a hospital. This certainly cannot enable top management to be in control of its quality management system and top management would be depriving itself of a most valuable management tool.

Extraordinary management review meetings may, of course, be called at any time by top management, but the standard agenda need not be used on such occasions.

The management representative will play a leading role in the preparations for the meetings and in the ensuing discussions.

Management review meetings must be recorded. The customary method is by means of minutes that include the findings of the reviews, the actions to be taken and the names of persons responsible for carrying through such actions by specified dates.

The revised standard identifies items for inclusion in the agenda of management review meetings (see clause 5.6.2) and through the output clause (see clause 5.6.3) requires decisions and corresponding actions to be identified. Well organized hospitals already do this through a comprehensive agenda, and proper minutes of meetings in which decisions are recorded with accompanying actions and dates for completion.

Review input (ISO 9001, clause 5.6.2)

This clause lists items that must be included in any management reviews:

(a) follow-up actions from previous management reviews;

(b) results of audits;

(c) improvements in patient processes and achievements in quality of life of patients;

(d) status of preventive and corrective actions;

(e) patient feedback (patient complaints and patient satisfaction surveys);

(f) recommendations for improvement;

(g) changes that could affect the quality management system.

Review output (ISO 9001, clause 5.6.3)

The outputs from the management review must include decisions and actions related to:

(a) improvement in the effectiveness of the quality management system and its processes;

(b) any changes likely to improve the quality of life of patients (advances in diagnosis; therapy, etc.);

(c) resource needs.

A typical agenda for a management review meeting

1. Apologies for absence;
2. Approval of the minutes of the previous management review meeting;
3. Matters arising from the previous minutes, not covered by the agenda below;
4. Internal audits: schedule; results of audits; corrective and preventive actions;
5. External audits/surveillances by certification body;
6. Performance of processes;
7. Nonconformities: corrective and preventive actions;
8. Patient feedback:
   - patient complaints; corrective actions; preventive actions;
   - monitoring of patient satisfaction;
9. Review of quality objectives;
10. Purchasing; suppliers' and subcontractors' lists;
11. Human resources:
    - competence requirements;
    - training needs;
    - evaluation of training;
    - skills testing;
12. Analysis of data;
13. Changes that could affect the quality management system;
14. Review of quality policy on a systematic basis (and as and when deemed necessary);
15. Continual improvements in the effectiveness of the quality management system;
16. Suggestions for improvements in the effectiveness of the processes, i.e. major and lower-level processes, attached notes;
17. Future resource needs;
18. Any other business;
19. Date of next meeting.

NOTE Time might not permit all the items on the agenda to be addressed at one meeting. Those not addressed can be given some preference at the subsequent meeting.

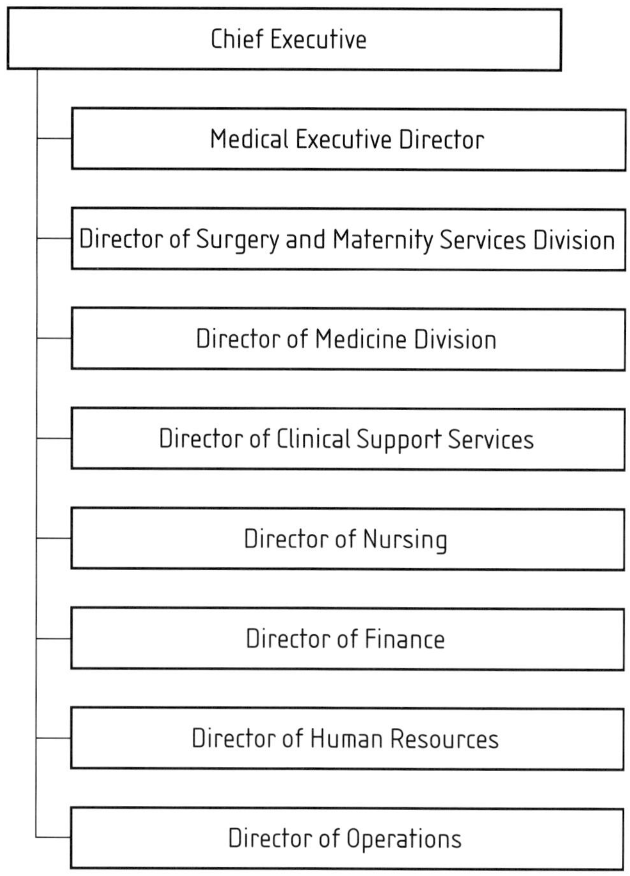

Figure 5.1 An organization chart

Chapter 6:
Resource management (clause 6)

Provision of resources (ISO 9001, clause 6.1)

Resources can be classified as: human resources, physical resources (i.e. hardware and equipment), the infrastructure and the work environment. All contribute in their different ways towards helping a hospital to achieve its overall goals and specific objectives.

Management must determine and provide the resources needed to implement and maintain the quality management system with a focus on continual improvement in the effectiveness of the quality management system in order to enhance patient satisfaction.

Management must also determine and provide the resources needed to enhance patient satisfaction, by helping clinicians to improve the quality of the lives of patients and to enable other staff to provide all the other services in connection with patient care.

Human resources (ISO 9001, clause 6.2)

General (ISO 9001, clause 6.2.1)

All employees whose duties and responsibilities might have a bearing on the quality of patient care in hospitals must be competent in the tasks that they have to carry out, as determined by their relevant education, training, skills and experience.

Competence, awareness and training (ISO 9001, clause 6.2.2)

Management must determine the necessary competences required for all personnel performing activities that have a bearing on the quality of patient care in hospitals.

In hospitals, many appointments can be made only on the basis of specific qualifications and training specified by professional bodies and the associated perceived competences associated with such qualifications and training. In those cases in which competence has been found wanting, perhaps because of an untoward incident, some kind of training or other actions may then be necessary in order to be certain that staff do have the previously defined competences.

In other posts in which a professional body is not involved, staff are appointed on the basis that a person has the necessary competences to perform the required tasks. If in practice this proves not to be the case, training should be offered to raise the competences of individuals to the necessary levels. A failure to attain the requirement competences, for whatever reason, means that the person must be redeployed on less demanding tasks, or have his/her employment terminated.

There are clearly many alternative and parallel routes for staff to achieve the necessary competences. For instance, each year a hospital can ask employees to undertake a self-appraisal using a prescribed form. Afterwards, employees are subjected to an appraisal, which is conducted in a prescribed manner by a more senior member of staff. Both the completed prescribed forms are held as confidential quality records. When management has to find people with specific competences such records on appraisals are invaluable. Even if there is nobody with the required competences, the appraisals might well enable someone to be chosen for training in order to achieve the required competences.

Once a person has been chosen, suitable training is given in a particular task or activity. Any training must be evaluated to determine whether the actions taken have been effective in making an employee competent in the clearly defined tasks.

All employees, whatever their status in the hospital, are made aware of the relevance and importance of the work that they are doing in contributing towards achieving the quality objectives of the hospital (see clause 5.4.1).

Appropriate records are maintained on all staff in terms of education, qualifications, training, experience, competency skills, as well as the evaluation records of any training courses undertaken. These are maintained as records (see clause 4.2.4).

Infrastructure (ISO 9001, clause 6.3)

Management needs to determine, provide and maintain the infrastructure needed to be able to diagnose and treat patients so that the needs and expectations of patients are satisfied within the accepted limitations of modern health care. These evidently include:

(a) appropriate buildings, wards, diagnostic and treatment areas, operating theatres, laboratories and associated facilities;

(b) diagnostic and therapeutic equipment, including up-to-date software;

(c) the necessary supporting services such as cleaners and communications services. Some of these might be outsourced.

Work environment (ISO 9001, clause 6.4)

The hospital has to determine the work environment that is needed to enable patients to have an acceptable environment whilst they are in hospital undergoing treatment or surgery.

The hospital also has to ensure that all employees work in a generally acceptable environment that is conducive to encouraging employees to give their best in terms of patient care. Such factors include:

a) safety of individuals (staff and patients);

b) ergonomics of working;

c) appropriate lighting levels;

d) appropriate temperature and humidity levels;

e) acceptable noise levels;

f) acceptable levels of cleanliness and hygiene;

g)) minimum pollution levels;

h) provision of appropriate protective equipment.

Many of these factors are the subject of legislation, regulation or codes of practice. The hospital management must ensure that appropriate controls are in place to ensure that the planned work environments are maintained.

Chapter 7:
Product realization (clause 7)

Planning of product realization (ISO 9001, clause 7.1)

Product realization is the term used to encompass all of those activities between establishing a patient's needs and attempting to achieve an improved quality of life for the patient.

A quality plan for achieving an improved quality of life for patients, whenever possible, is the result of deliberations on what needs to be done in a systematic manner in order to achieve that objective for all patients. The documentation resulting from such planning can be in whatever form is most suitable for the hospital's mode of operations. In the case of a simple diagnosis and treatment, a few comments/instructions in a patient's case notes might be all that is required as a quality plan. In more complex cases, the quality plan might require much more than simply just a few words in the patient case notes: back-up reports, test results, X-ray films and ultrasound scans, on which a diagnosis is based and a treatment plan is determined.

A patient's treatment plan must identify every activity that is necessary to achieve an improved quality of life for the patient. All processes that are an integral part of the quality management system of the hospital need to be identified (see clause 4.1). These include the first-level processes and any other supplementary processes. Appropriate documentation needs to be created (e.g. lower-level processes and appended notes) as is considered necessary, to control all the processes. The treatment plan must include measurable quality objectives that are set at relevant functions and levels within the hospital (see clause 5.4.1). Human and physical resources specific to the needs of the patient must be identified. Any patient monitoring, inspection and test activities required for patient diagnosis and treatment must be identified. Some of the monitoring and measuring devices might need to be calibrated and their calibrations linked to international standards. Specific criteria for patient diagnosis and treatment might have to be established for patient care associated with the general criterion of an improved quality of life for all patients. Questions have to be answered on how the improved quality of life of a patient will be validated within the limitations of any practicalities. In many cases this will be simple, but in some cases it will not be.

If a hospital decides to outsource any process that can have a bearing on the quality of patient care, the hospital must ensure appropriate control over such processes. Examples of outsourcing may include use of an independent pharmacy or, in the case of private hospitals, independent surgeons.

Decisions are required on the records that will be kept. Such records (see clause 4.2.4) will provide objective evidence that patient care has followed the relevant process, apart from changes deemed necessary and initiated by the clinician responsible for patient care.

If planned changes to the quality management system are implemented, the integrity of the quality management system must be maintained [see clause 5.4.2(b)].

Any patient plan should be structured so that everyone is made aware of the need continually to improve the effectiveness of the quality management system, and suggestions for such improvements will always be welcomed through recognized channels by top management.

Customer-related processes (ISO 9001, clause 7.2)

Determination of requirements related to the product (ISO 9001, clause 7.2.1)

The needs of patients are paramount. They can be summed up by the desire of patients to have an improved quality of life on leaving the hospital. In the UK the government publishes guidelines to hospitals using guidance from organizations such as NICE and NSF (see Appendix 3).

Review of requirements related to the product (ISO 9001, clause 7.2.2)

The clinicians responsible for the diagnosis and treatment of patients must review patient requirements before embarking upon treatment of patients. In many cases such reviews are simple, in that the senior clinician (usually a consultant) decides what actions need to be taken. In more complex cases several specialist consultants might be involved in such reviews. The outcome of any review process must be that the needs of patients are clearly defined and any subsequent follow-up actions are fully documented (see clause 4.2.4).

If the needs of patients are changed, all relevant documentation must be amended and the relevant personnel advised accordingly.

Customer communication (ISO 9001, clause 7.2.3)

The requirement for hospitals to identify the channels of communication with their patients and to adhere strictly to such channels are common sense requirements that are already common practice in many hospitals. The revised standard requires management to determine and implement effective channels of communication between the hospital and its patients on all matters in relation to the care of patients.

Patient feedback can be either verbal or written. It can be reactive or proactive. Patient complaints must be dealt with in a systematic manner (see Chapter 8). An example of a proactive case is the monitoring of patient satisfaction (see clause 8.2.1). Whatever the nature of the feedback from patients, arrangements must be in place for dealing with it in a systematic manner (see PC 104).

Design and development (ISO 9001, clause 7.3)

The design and development clause can be excluded from the quality management system for hospitals. The justification for this is dealt with in Chapter 9.

Purchasing (ISO 9001, clause 7.4)

Purchasing process (ISO 9001, clause 7.4.1)

In the UK there is a considerable amount of central purchasing and a hospital has little direct control over such purchases. If free to do so, a hospital must ensure that a purchased product or service conforms to specified purchase requirements. A hospital must evaluate potential suppliers and subcontractors on this basis. There are many ways in which this can be done, for example:

- by means of questionnaires;
- visits by the supplier or subcontractor to learn about the hospital in general;
- conducting an audit on those parts of the supplier or subcontractor that are of particular interest;
- by placing a trial order, if this is feasible;
- by asking for the opinions of others.

Hospitals can choose the ways in which suppliers and subcontractors are evaluated, but the criteria for evaluation, selection and any necessary re-evaluation must be defined.

The results of evaluations/selections and any subsequent follow-up actions must be recorded and held as records (see clause 4.2.4).

In practical terms, after evaluation and selection many hospitals generate an approved list of suppliers and subcontractors. Some also have a temporary list. The temporary list includes suppliers and subcontractors that are being used and may be transferred to the approved list in due course. Transfer can take place after a satisfactory track record has been established, after a second-party audit has been conducted, or by whatever other means is considered appropriate, to determine whether transfer to the approved list can be made.

Some hospitals also have a non-approved list, which include suppliers and subcontractors that have not met the hospital's required standards. The non-approved list reminds all employees that orders must not be placed with suppliers and subcontractors on that list.

The performance of chosen suppliers should be reviewed on a regular basis and the lists should be updated as necessary. Evidence of updating should be available. Suppliers and subcontractors that provide products and/or services that are unlikely to have any bearing on the quality of the product and/or service provided by the hospital need not be subjected to the same scrutiny.

Some hospitals find that, as a result of implementing the requirements of the standard, an opportunity is provided to decrease the number of suppliers and subcontractors with consequential savings in administration.

Purchasing information (ISO 9001, clause 7.4.2)

Purchase orders and associated documents need to contain all the information that a supplier or a subcontractor will need in order to satisfy the hospital's requirements. Any associated documentation referred to in the purchase order will stress any conditional requirements of placing the order. Verbal orders always need to be followed by documented purchase orders and associated documentation so that both parties are fully aware of what has been ordered and under what conditions.

Most hospitals clearly describe on their purchase orders (and any associated documents) what is required and have designated levels of authority to review and approve such orders. This is not a very onerous requirement. In simple cases it is implicit that the person signing the order has, as a minimum, looked at the order and given an approval of adequacy, as would be the case for standard off-the-shelf items, which are unlikely to pose problems. However, in the case of complex orders for a manufactured product, or a sophisticated service, the hospital might have to impose some sort of checklist, each section of which would have to be signed off by named signatories, before a final signature is added by a purchasing manager, or in the case of very big orders, by a director of the hospital. Each hospital must decide what is appropriate for its own circumstances within the remit of the standard.

Verification of purchased product (ISO 9001, clause 7.4.3)

The nature and extent of the controls applied to a selected supplier or subcontractor will be dependent on the effect the purchased product, or service provided, has on the hospital's processes and on the possible quality of life of patients. Some purchased products or services that are regarded by the hospital as being crucial to the success of its operations are likely to be subjected to strict controls. Other products or services that are much less important will be subject to less stringent controls.

The activities necessary for verification of purchased product must be identified and implemented. The associated documents referred to above might specify that a supplier provides a test certificate, in which case the supplier is confirming that the product meets the required specification. In other cases an accredited calibration certificate might be required. In many cases, if the supplier has an established track record with the hospital, the verification of product on receipt at the hospital will be minimal. With a new supplier, the hospital might well impose strict verification processes, which will have been identified in advance and implemented on receipt of goods.

If verification is to be performed by the hospital at the supplier's premises, the hospital will specify the intended verification arrangements and method of product release in the purchasing documents (i.e. in the order or contract document). The purchasing document should state how verification would be conducted. For instance, in the case of manufactured products, will there be 100% testing, batch testing or sampling? In the case of a service, what specified items are to be checked, or is random testing to be used? Finally, the purchasing document should state what acceptance criteria are to be used and who is to be responsible for release of product to the hospital, or acceptance of the service to be provided for the hospital.

Production and service provision (ISO 9001, clause 7.5)

Control of production and service provision (ISO 9001, clause 7.5.1)

The major process in a hospital is the diagnosis and treatment of patients. This is done in a systematic way, as explained in PD 101. The first step is common to all patients on entering hospital. Its purpose is to collect basic information about the general state of a patient and to carry out simple tests on the patient. What follows are more detailed and often highly technical investigations to determine the precise cause of a problem. Each investigation is usually done without reference to other specialists, unless it is necessary to refer to others. Treatment then follows, which can be in the form of drugs or surgery. The outcomes are recorded at each stage in the patient's case notes which accompany the patient at all times. Finally, discharge takes place, with provision for follow up by the patient's GP or at out-patient clinics, or both.

All major and lower-level processes must be adequately controlled with one objective in mind, namely an improved quality of life of the patient, whenever possible. Appropriate documentation must be in place for patient care. Appropriate documentation must also be available that will allow all the processes to be carried out in an effective and satisfactory manner. Adequate equipment must be provided, including any monitoring and measuring devices that are necessary for any monitoring and measurements that are required on patients. The formal discharge of patients from a hospital can be conducted only with the approval of the clinician who has been responsible for patient care.

Post-hospital care should be specified prior to discharge from hospital. All the above activities should have been planned before patient care begins. The controls should have ensured that planned provisions have been adhered to in all respects.

Validation of processes for production and service provision (ISO 9001, clause 7.5.2)

In general, hospitals are able to demonstrate that the results of patient care can be validated by measurements, monitoring or other investigations, to prove that the planned output, namely the expected improvement in the patient's condition has been achieved (or not achieved, as is sometimes the case in hospital work). When a patient is given medication, a clinician is able to determine whether it has achieved the desired result. If it has been only partially successful the clinician may make changes to the medication in the hope of achieving a better patient outcome. In surgical cases there are several indirect methods, e.g. radiology, of determining whether surgery has been successful. At worst, if the outcome for a patient has not been as planned, operating again is a possibility, either immediately, in cases of a serious failure, or in the near future. It would therefore appear that, as far as direct patient care is concerned, this clause could be justifiably excluded since it is always possible to validate the outcomes of direct patient care.

The clause cannot completely, however, be excluded from the quality management system of a hospital because of at least one activity that takes place within hospitals that is indirectly associated with patient care, namely, sterilization of surgical gowns, drapes and surgical instruments. A hospital must validate any service processes when subsequent measuring or monitoring cannot readily or economically verify the resulting output. These processes are referred to as process validation in ISO 9001:2000 (they were referred to as special processes in ISO 9001:1994) and they must be continually monitored and controlled by specially trained staff. Sterilization is one such classic example.

In all such cases, proving what has been achieved results in the output being damaged or completely ruined. For instance, opening a particular sterilized package to check whether sterilization has actually been achieved results in a package that has to be sterilized again before it can be used as intended. Instead, strict measures are usually in place, such as specially trained practitioners, special equipment and devices, and processes/procedures that have to be followed rigidly to ensure that the planned results are in fact achieved.

Validation arrangements must include, as applicable:

- the qualification of the processes, i.e. defined criteria for review and approval of the processes;
- approval of equipment and qualification/competence of personnel;

- use of specific methods and procedures;
- requirements for records (see clause 4.2.4);
- revalidation, following repeat of a process.

Identification and traceability (ISO 9001, clause 7.5.3)

Identification

The onus is placed on a hospital to decide how best to identify patients uniquely. Whenever monitoring and measurements are made during patient care, the hospital must identify the status of the patient care process at a given time (see clause 8.2.4) to establish that the process of patient care can proceed to the next stage.

It is advisable to maintain records of any identification data that are used (see procedure PC 102 and clause 4.2.4).

Traceability

If traceability is explicitly required on any items or processes, the hospital must control and record the unique identification of individual items, batches of items or special processes, as is considered appropriate.

Whilst traceability is essential in some cases, it can also be useful in much less onerous circumstances. For example, in the case of a cleaning service, a hospital often considers it useful to be able to identify which cleaners did what on certain dates and, thereby, provide full traceability on the service provided.

It is advisable to maintain records on all traceability data used (see PC 102 and clause 4.2.4).

Customer property (ISO 9001, clause 7.5.4)

General

The hospital must ensure that due care is exercised with patient property. Any confidential information provided by a patient must be respected as such. A hospital is expected to communicate immediately with a patient in the event of untoward happenings with the patient's property.

Lost/damaged/unsuitable patient property

Any patient property that is lost, or damaged, must be reported to the patient. A record of the loss, or damage, must be made and maintained.

Preservation of product (ISO 9001, clause 7.5.5)

General

As explained earlier, the product of a hospital is the improved quality of life of the patient. Every effort must be made at all times whilst a patient is in hospital to ensure that the quality of life of the patient is not allowed to deteriorate in any way.

Identification

As explained in the commentary to clause 7.5.3, the onus is placed on the hospital to decide how best to uniquely identify patients.

Handling

The onus is on the hospital to devise methods of handling patients that ensure that patients are not hurt or injured whilst they are being lifted or handled in any way.

Packaging

Not applicable.

Storage

Not applicable.

Protection

A hospital is expected to provide protection for its patients at all times from malicious damage, sexual assault, etc. whilst within the confines of the hospital. A hospital is expected to provide protection of stock against damage, theft, etc.

(In the event of a patient dying, certain measures must be in place to ensure the remains of the deceased are treated in a dignified manner. Access to the mortuary must be properly controlled so that corpses are protected and accorded a secure resting place.)

Preservation

A hospital must ensure that all patients are adequately cared for at all times and are secure from assault, etc.

Delivery

Hospitals often have to move patients within the confines of a hospital. Sometimes patients have to be transferred to other hospitals for treatment or care. Due care must be taken to ensure that this is always done in a safe manner.

Control of monitoring and measuring devices (ISO 9001, clause 7.6)

Clinicians decide for themselves what measurements are needed in connection with patient care. In many cases the accuracy of any measurements with a given measuring device is unimportant and there is no need to have such devices calibrated. This does not mean that routine maintenance is unimportant. For instance, traditional sphygmomanometers need to undergo maintenance, because of the wear and tear that they experience in frequent use, but they do not have to be calibrated since they provide only a crude measurement of patient blood pressure and are subject to variations in human measuring errors.

It is also important to differentiate between measurement and monitoring.

Monitoring

If measuring devices are being used to monitor a patient's condition, the monitoring might be taking place continuously. Such measuring devices immediately identify any untoward changes that are occurring so that appropriate action can be taken immediately. If the changes or trends are taking place slowly, they give early warning of problems.

Monitoring, using measuring devices, is not always done continuously. It might be done continually, i.e. from time to time, as determined by a protocol or as determined by the clinician responsible for the care of a particular patient.

Monitoring does not always involve measuring devices. For instance, the standard requires a hospital to monitor patient satisfaction. This can be done without measuring devices (see commentary to clause 8.2.1).

Measurement

There is little doubt about what is meant by measurement. Measurement is associated with, for example, determination of a number, length, area, volume, time, speed, velocity, acceleration or weight.

The need for monitoring and measurements

As already mentioned, clinicians decide what monitoring and measurements are necessary to ensure that a patient's diagnosis and subsequent treatment are satisfactory. This, in turn, determines what monitoring and measuring devices are needed to provide evidence of conformity of patient care to previously determined requirements (see clause 7.2.1). All measuring and monitoring devices must be used and controlled so that they are capable of making measurements to the required degree of accuracy. As already stated, in the case of many devices used in hospitals, calibration of measuring devices is unnecessary.

However, when it is decided that measuring devices need to be calibrated to ensure that measurements meet the required accuracy, calibration must be done properly. This means that measuring devices must:

(a) be calibrated or verified at specified intervals, or prior to use, against measurement standards traceable to international or national measurement standards; where no such standards exist, the basis used for calibration or verification must be recorded;

(b) be adjusted or readjusted as necessary;

(c) be identified to enable calibration status to be determined;

(d) be safeguarded from adjustments that would invalidate the measurement result;

(e) be protected from damage and deterioration during handling, maintenance and storage;

(f) have results of calibration and verification recorded and held as records.

Computer software used for measuring and monitoring of specified requirements must be checked prior to initial use, and re-checked at appropriate specified intervals, to ensure that it satisfies the intended application.

It should be noted that different devices need to be calibrated at different intervals. Some devices are not used very often and are more stable as a result. Devices that are used regularly and devices that are highly sensitive will need to be calibrated at more frequent intervals. The same applies to any device where the accuracy of the results is of very special significance.

External calibration

If a decision is made in favour of external calibration, the calibration can be carried out by an accredited calibration laboratory, which has been accredited by the United Kingdom Accreditation Service (UKAS), by another similar national accreditation body, or by a non-accredited calibration body. ISO 9001:2000, like the 1994 standard, does not require a UKAS (or equivalent) calibration laboratory to be used. Both standards do, however, require that calibration can be traced to international or national measurement standards.

Internally calibrated equipment

When a hospital has a lot of equipment that needs to be calibrated and has suitably qualified staff available, it may decide to calibrate its own equipment using carefully selected externally calibrated equipment as reference standards.

It is good practice to have a work instruction available for each kind of equipment that is to be calibrated internally, to ensure that all relevant matters are addressed and that the steps to be taken in the calibration process are clearly defined.

Registers and calibration logs

It is common practice to establish and maintain calibration registers and calibration logs for all calibrated equipment. All such registers and logs become part of the hospital's records (see PC 102 and clause 4.2.4).

Identification of devices

All calibrated equipment (whether externally or internally calibrated) should be uniquely identified by whatever means is practical. It is common practice for each piece of calibrated equipment to have a label affixed which states:

- the unique identification number or code for the equipment;
- the date when calibration took place;
- the date when recalibration is due;
- the initials of the person responsible for calibration.

A label, which includes the date of recalibration, enables the user to check that the equipment has not passed that recalibration date without recalibration having taken place.

In very unusual circumstances it is impossible to place such a label on calibrated equipment. In such circumstances, a unique identification number can be engraved on the equipment, the equipment can be marked with an indelible pencil, or a very small sticker can be used, which gives the equipment a unique number. Such arrangements enable the equipment to be referred back to the calibration records.

If a piece of equipment has a calibration label affixed to it, it means that the equipment, when tested on a specific date and under agreed specified conditions, was functioning in accordance with its specification and within the specified limits of accuracy.

The registers and calibration logs should show the normal locations of calibrated devices so that in the event that a label is detached from a device its unique identification and calibration status can be traced through a process of elimination.

Fitness for use

This is a common sense requirement. Some equipment is less susceptible to damage than other equipment. The hospital must exercise appropriate controls to ensure that, as far as possible, accuracy and fitness for use is maintained.

Tampering with calibrations

In most cases calibrated equipment cannot unintentionally and easily be put out of calibration. Nevertheless, the hospital must take all reasonable measures to ensure that any intentional tampering is positively discouraged, if not made virtually impossible.

Out-of-calibration equipment

When a piece of calibrated equipment is suspected of being out of calibration, it must be removed immediately from use.

The question then arises as to how long the device might have been out of calibration and what are the possible consequences of the use of the device on patients diagnosed or treated earlier. In such circumstances, top management of the hospital is required to make a judgement on the effect of any possible adverse consequences on the patients and then take appropriate action, such as the recall of patients. The decisions and the actions taken must be fully documented (see PC 102 and clause 4.2.4).

New equipment

There is a popular misconception that it can be assumed that a piece of new equipment is accurate within its specification. If a manufacturer provides a valid certificate of calibration then this must be true. Similarly, a carefully scrutinized test certificate from a manufacturer would increase confidence in a new product. However, if there are any doubts about the accuracy of a device and a specified accuracy is crucial to patient diagnosis or treatment, it is prudent to have the device re-checked carefully.

Chapter 8:
Measurement, analysis and improvement (clause 8)

General (ISO 9001, clause 8.1)

Management must plan and implement monitoring, measurement, analysis and improvement processes needed to:

- ensure conformity of the quality management system with the requirements of the standard;
- demonstrate conformity of hospital processes that have the objective of improving the quality of life of patients;
- continually improve the effectiveness of the quality management system of the hospital.

All data from monitoring and measurements must be collated and analysed. The monitoring and measurements made during a patient process might enable appropriate changes to be made to ensure the continuing ability of each step in a patient process to achieve its intended purpose. Monitoring and measurements also enable checks to be made on whether the final product, namely an 'improved quality of life' of the patient, emerges at the end of the patient process.

The data collected and analysed can also provide ongoing information as a foundation for possible changes to continually improve the effectiveness of the quality management system of the hospital.

In planning any monitoring and measuring activities, due consideration must always be given to deciding how the data collected are to be used.

Monitoring and measurement (ISO 9001, clause 8.2)

Customer satisfaction (ISO 9001, clause 8.2.1)

A hospital is required to monitor (not measure) patient satisfaction in a proactive manner to determine whether patient satisfaction has been achieved. Each hospital can determine how it monitors patient satisfaction, although the methods used for obtaining and using the information have to be determined and explained. The monitoring must focus on patient perceptions of whether the hospital has met patient requirements (see clause 7.2.1).

Information on patient satisfaction can be obtained in a number of ways. Some examples follow.

By direct communication with patients

(a) by patient satisfaction questionnaires;

The standard method of obtaining information from patients regarding their satisfaction is for a hospital to issue a form to patients and ask them to complete and return it, either before or after leaving hospital. Such forms can vary enormously in their complexity, but the more complex the form the less likely it is to be completed.

Although collection of information or feedback from patients might be considered to have been reasonably successful, the analysis of such data needs to be undertaken carefully to provide a true measure of a hospital's success in satisfying the needs of patients. Any analysis highlights the importance of asking the right questions and often, after receipt of the first batch of completed questionnaires, changes will need to be made to the questionnaire to improve the feedback from patients. Hospitals should keep their questionnaires very simple with only a few carefully thought out questions. Large hospitals can produce questionnaires that have many more questions. The answers can be entered into a computer and computer analysis is clearly helpful in obtaining indicators of patient satisfaction.

The serial analyses of patient satisfaction questionnaires should be considered at management reviews when weaknesses and strengths will be highlighted and perhaps new quality objectives can be set for the ensuing period.

(b) by telephone enquiries;

Another way is to telephone a given percentage of patients who have used the hospital in some way or other during the previous week or month.

Secondary sources of information related to patient satisfaction

(c) by independent investigations;

In the UK one such source is the *Which?* reports published by the Consumers' Association and media investigations such as the BBC 'Watchdog' programmes. Both of these sources often focus on specific services provided by hospitals that have resulted in intense dissatisfaction by a number of patients.

(d) by media reports;

Journalists often focus on hospitals or on individuals who get things wrong or do things badly, and they can highlight public dissatisfaction. Documentary television programmes are produced to highlight difficulties experienced by patients.

Such secondary sources of patient satisfaction/dissatisfaction will probably be applicable perhaps to only one hospital. All hospitals should be aware of adverse reports so that the problems highlighted are not allowed to occur in other hospitals.

Relying on the number of patient complaints to give an indication of patient satisfaction is unlikely to give the complete picture. A relatively small number of complaints received and recorded may be only the tip of an iceberg as far as patient dissatisfaction is concerned.

In all cases of patient dissatisfaction, there may be various degrees of incompetence of individuals and/or incompetence of management. The revised standard appears to recognize this by placing more emphasis on the responsibilities of management and, for the first time, requires evidence that training of employees has resulted in individuals becoming more competent, or that they have achieved new competences as a result of their training (see clause 6.2.2).

Internal audit (ISO 9001, clause 8.2.2)

Internal audits have to be carried out at planned intervals to determine whether the quality management system:

- conforms to the requirements of the standard;
- has been effectively implemented and is being maintained;
- has identified and is conforming to the planned arrangements for the processes that have been identified by the clinicians in their attempts to improve the quality of life of patients.

The requirement regarding conformance with the requirements of the standard is new in that in ISO 9001:1994, internal auditors had to verify only whether quality activities and related results complied with planned arrangements and also to determine the effectiveness of the quality system. In other words, internal audits were used to focus on compliance with the hospital's protocols, procedures and work instructions, as well as on the effectiveness of the quality system, but not on conformance with the requirements of the standard.

There is one other important change. ISO 9001:1994 states that only personnel independent of those having direct responsibility for the activity being audited must carry out audits. ISO 9001:2000 is different. It merely states that auditors must not audit their own work.

A mandatory procedure (see PC 103) is required on internal auditing that defines:

- the responsibilities and requirements for planning and conducting audits;
- how results will be reported;
- how records will be kept and maintained.

With ISO 9001:2000, the main focus of internal auditing is on the patient process and the resulting outcomes. Auditors are expected to follow a patient process from the time a patient is referred to a hospital to the time that he or she leaves the hospital. In working through a major process, pauses in the steps forward will be inevitable and frequent, during which time lower-level processes and attached notes may have to be checked. These, in turn, may result in examination of compliance with other documents associated with a major process, e.g. calibrations. Thus, some compliance auditing will still continue to be necessary.

An audit program, or audit schedule (see FM 121), must be prepared that covers all the areas applicable to the audit. Once a hospital's major processes have been clearly identified, all the audits associated with such processes can be planned. The schedule must identify the frequency of such audits based on the status and importance of various activities. The schedule of internal audits should be flexible and changes will be inevitable as the results of earlier audits become available.

Auditing is both an art and a science (for further information see *ISO 9001 Quality Systems Auditing* [8]). Internal auditing must be carried out by auditors who have been trained in the techniques of auditing. Training can be conducted by the organization's experienced auditors, or it can be done externally by attendance on approved courses. Any good auditor can conduct an internal audit in any circumstances. Less experienced auditors would benefit from the preparation of audit questions before an audit is conducted (see FM 123). The questions need not be rigidly adhered to. They can be regarded as starter questions that will lead on to further questioning if an auditor feels that there is a need to pursue matters in greater detail.

A well-designed Nonconformity or Observation Form (see FM 124), included in the procedure is recommended for use during internal audits. This will include as a minimum:

- a section for defining the nonconformity (or observation);
- when and where it was found (i.e. which department);
- the corrective actions agreed to be taken, by whom and by when (see clause 8.5.2).

The form should include space for preventive action to be recorded, if this is deemed necessary (see clause 8.5.3). Another section requires verification of the corrective action (and, perhaps, preventive action) by the management representative or another designated person.

The new focus on processes will mean that internal audits are likely to take much more time and skill than would be the case if an auditor were merely checking for compliance with one or more, perhaps isolated, procedures. Auditing should become much more interesting and more meaningful because of its direct link with the reasons why a hospital exists. Moreover, in discussions with auditees, it should provide opportunities for considering ways in which changes might be made to the major process (and any supplementary processes) so that it can be improved.

In the case of a diagnostic investigation, consider a radiological department (see process diagram, PD 102). An auditor would follow the trail of the patient from the time they were admitted into the department (i.e. via appointment, referral or emergency admission) until the completion of the diagnostic process. The outcome would be the examination of the X-ray by a radiologist. An ISO 9001 internal auditor who was not a radiologist would not be expected to decide whether an X-ray has been interpreted correctly. The X-ray and the report on the X-ray become part of the diagnostic process records and, once the patient leaves hospital, the X-ray becomes a quality management system record, carefully stored and protected from damage, as has always been the case, for possible future use. If wrong interpretations of X-rays come to light at a later stage, other independent radiological experts carry out further checks. Such happenings do occur as exemplified by a number of cases in the public domain in recent times in connection with breast screening services.

All hospital employees should realize that auditing should be looked upon in a positive manner. Its purpose is to make things better for all concerned, but especially for the patients. The impartial auditing process enables any shortcomings in a process to be highlighted and affords an excellent opportunity to make changes for continuing improvements in the effectiveness of the quality management system. Any improvements will affect the overall efficiency of the hospital with consequential benefits to patients. Maximum benefits accrue from internal auditing when there is openness, integrity and responsibility, as explained under corporate governance (see Appendix 2).

The findings and follow-up actions arising from internal audits are a key item on the agenda of management review meetings, which includes the effectiveness of any corrective and preventive actions.

Monitoring and measurement of processes (ISO 9001, clause 8.2.3)

All major processes must be monitored and measured, as and when deemed necessary, in such ways that the output of a major process will focus on an end result that is intended to result in an improved quality of life for a patient. All monitoring and measurements are done with the intention of confirming the continuing ability of each major process to achieve the specified requirements at each stage of a major process. In the event that requirements are not being met, nonconformities should be raised. The nonconformity form used is essentially the same as that used in connection with internal audits.

Lower-level processes also need to be a monitored in the same way. Lower-level processes do not necessarily impact directly on major processes when, for instance, a failure to carry them out might not prevent such processes from proceeding to an improved quality of life for a patient. One example of a lower-level process would be calibration of measuring and test equipment. If recalibration of such equipment does not take place at the scheduled time, it does not mean that the equipment was necessarily inaccurate at the time it was used in a major process.

The quality management system should have processes in place to report nonconformities to top management, who, in turn, should have in place a process to report serious incidents to the National Institute of Clinical Excellence (NICE).

Monitoring and measurement of product (ISO 9001, clause 8.2.4)

Monitoring and measuring the quality of life of a patient must take place at appropriate stages of a major process to ensure that the planned treatment is being followed (see clause 7.1). Evidence of conformity with accepted criteria must be documented and finally authority for discharge of a patient must be recorded (see clause 4.2.4). Such documentation becomes part of the hospital's records.

Patients must not be discharged until there is documented evidence that all specified monitoring and measurements have been satisfactorily completed (see clause 7.1) and approval is given by a senior clinician, namely, a senior house officer, registrar or consultant. Housemen and nurses can discharge patients on the explicit instructions of a senior clinician when objective evidence becomes available that specific conditions in the patient have been attained. A discharge summary is created that includes a follow-up appointment date. (In exceptional circumstances, patients might choose to discharge themselves.)

Control of nonconforming product (ISO 9001, clause 8.3)

In manufacturing, products do not always satisfy the requirements of customers and in the service industry what has been agreed is not always provided. Likewise, patient care in hospitals sometimes fails to satisfy expectations.

Hospitals are complex organizations but their planned outputs are always the same, namely, an improved quality of life of the patient. Any failure to achieve an improved quality of life for a patient might arise because what was planned for a particular patient was not carried out satisfactorily, or simply because a patient has not responded to the planned treatment as expected for reasons unknown at the time. In extreme circumstances, it could also be that the planned treatment has resulted in the deterioration of a patient's quality of life. Ideally, in such circumstances a clinician would review his/her treatment plan to try and improve the quality of life of their patient in a different way.

Procedure PC 104 might be applicable when patients do not respond to treatment. The scope of PC 104 states:

> The failure of a patient to respond to treatment as expected is not to be regarded as a nonconformity since treatment of patients is not an exact science. However, the failure to give the correct amount of a drug (wrongly prescribed, or carelessness on the part of a clinician), or the wrong injection of a drug into the spine, as opposed to being injected into the venous system, is to be regarded as a nonconformity, and recorded as such.

In all cases where nonconformities arise, which could affect the quality of life of a patient, every effort should be made to identify and record the causes of nonconformities on appropriate nonconformity forms.

Top management must review all factual information on nonconformities. The regular management reviews are intended to be the focus of such discussions. Unplanned management reviews can, of course, be called at any time. Clinical nonconformities will require action as soon as a suspected nonconformity arises. In some cases when nonconformity becomes known, top management must decide whether the same nonconformity might have been occurring for some time. If this is the case, it means that appropriate action must be taken regarding the consequences, or potential effects, of the nonconformity. It may be necessary to recall some patients for further investigations.

Only after full investigation should a clinical nonconformity form be signed off by a senior management person confirming the investigation has been completed and appropriate actions taken.

Top management should be in a better position to manage nonconformities if:

(a) nonconformities are identified;

(b) the reasons for each nonconformity are identified;

(c) appropriate corrective actions are taken; and

(d) all relevant information [such as (a), (b) and (c)] is fully documented.

Analysis of data (ISO 9001, clause 8.4)

A hospital has to determine what data, when collected, collated and analysed, can be used to demonstrate the suitability and effectiveness of its quality management system and show how such analyses can be used to achieve continual improvement in the effectiveness of the quality management system (see clause 8.5.1).

Data can be obtained from any relevant sources in addition to the four sources specifically named in the standard. These are:

(a) the characteristics and trends of patient processes and patient outcomes, including opportunities for preventive action;

(b) achievements in improving the quality of life of patients (see clause 7.2.1);

(c) patient satisfaction (see clause 8.2.1);

(d) the performance of suppliers (including central purchasing).

Improvement (ISO 9001, clause 8.5)

Continual improvement (ISO 9001, clause 8.5.1)

The hospital must continually improve the effectiveness of its quality management system. This is a new explicit requirement that is repeated many times in ISO 9001.

Planning and striving for continual improvements in the effectiveness of the quality management system is to be achieved through the use of the quality policy, quality objectives, internal auditing, analysis of data, corrective and preventive actions and through management reviews.

The requirement for continual improvement in the effectiveness of the quality management system means that a hospital should always be striving to make changes that will result in improvements in the interests of efficiency and economy. In fact these are all the things that a good hospital should be doing in any case, irrespective of ISO 9001. Possible initiatives that might result in continual improvements in the effectiveness of a quality management system include:

- changes in management of a hospital;
- new resources (more competent people and better physical resources);
- improved monitoring and measurements during processes;
- better collection and analysis of data;
- new or improved technology.

Corrective action (ISO 9001, clause 8.5.2)

A hospital must take corrective action to eliminate the cause of nonconformities (discovered during internal audits, during processes, including clinical processes, and when the end result of a process is not a better quality of life for a patient) as well as in the case of patient complaints in order to prevent a reoccurrence.

Nonconformities

A corrective action procedure (see PC 105) is required for:

- reviewing nonconformities;
- determining the causes of nonconformities;
- evaluating the need for action to ensure that nonconformities do not reoccur;
- determining the corrective action needed;
- implementing the corrective action needed;
- recording the results of the corrective action taken (see clause 4.2.4);
- reviewing the corrective action taken.

As explained earlier, every nonconformity should be recorded on a prescribed nonconformity form by the person identifying the complaint or by a nominated person or persons. The form identifies the nonconformity and who identified it, and the date and time of identification. The form includes space to state the corrective action taken. The person who accepts responsibility for the corrective action should sign that part of the form. Finally, the prescribed form should only be signed off by a responsible person within the hospital, usually the management representative, when they are satisfied that the nonconformity has been satisfactorily dealt with from every point of view and that the actions taken have been completed in every respect and proved to be effective, or apparently so.

Nonconformity forms are systematically filed and presented at regular management reviews. One person, usually the management representative, provides a summary of events since the last management review meeting.

Corrective actions must always be appropriate to the impact of the problem encountered and the likelihood of it happening again. For example, a large amount of money should not be spent following a single nonconformity or a single complaint (provided the outcome has not been disastrous for a patient) when either is considered to be a one–off event with a very low probability of reoccurrence.

Patient complaints

There seems to be some doubt about what is meant by a patient complaint. A good guideline is that if anyone in a hospital feels that they should apologise to a patient, because the patient appears to be aggrieved by what has happened, or by what has not happened, then a complaint has been received. It may appear to be an unjustifiable complaint, but the patient evidently thinks otherwise so it is advisable to proceed cautiously and to promise to investigate the complaint without delay.

There must be a full investigation and response to patient complaints, whether they are verbal or written complaints. All patient complaints should be logged and dealt with in a systematic manner as detailed in the ISO 9001 mandatory procedure PC 105, corrective action. They should be dealt with immediately and in the case of a serious complaint, the details should be passed to the chief executive for immediate action. The first priority should be to investigate the complaint and correct what has allegedly gone wrong. Very often, an appropriate explanation and perhaps an apology is all that is necessary and the goodwill between the hospital and the patient is rapidly restored.

There is little difference in the ways in which nonconformities and complaints are dealt with, apart from the need for a quick response from the hospital in the case of a patient complaint. Management should look upon patient complaints in a positive manner. They should not be used to ostracize people. Complaints are an important management tool whereby lessons can be learned.

The absence of patient complaints must not lead to the assumption that all patients are entirely satisfied with a hospital. Some hospitals may not have a sufficiently accessible method of dealing with complaints. The introduction of a quality management system based on ISO 9001 will certainly ensure that this happens. All complaints, not just serious complaints, must be systematically recorded and dealt with promptly.

Since April 2002 a national system has been used in UK hospitals to deal with patient complaints (see Appendix 3: Patient Advisory and Liaison Service, PALS). The latest paper from the Department of Health [9] shows that there is still much to be done to establish an effective and acceptable method of dealing with patient complaints.

Preventive action (ISO 9001, clause 8.5.3)

Preventive action is action taken to prevent something that has happened in the past (nonconformities, patient complaints) from taking place again in the future. Another important kind of preventive action is action taken to prevent something from happening in the future that has not happened so far. A mandatory procedure is required on preventive actions (see PC 106).

Any preventive actions taken must be appropriate to the impact of the problem that has arisen. For instance, what is considered to be a one–off occurrence (assuming no serious patient outcome has occurred) should not result in enormous expenditure to prevent its reoccurrence. Similarly, a theoretical possibility of something occurring in the future might not justify considerable expense to reduce the probability of it happening. Thus, it might be decided in the case of a particular incident that no preventive action is to be taken.

Chapter 9:
Design and development: justifiable exclusions

Most people have no experience of design and development work. Those who have know that the design and development clause in ISO 9001:2000 is excellent. This clause is identical to clause 4.4 in ISO 9001:1994 standard, except that one part in the 1994 standard has been subsumed into one of the clauses in ISO 9001:2000.

People who have no experience of design and development work are advised to examine ISO 9001, clause 7.3 very carefully, sentence by sentence and also as an overall requirement.

ISO 9001, clause 7.3 contains the following clauses:

- 7.3.1 design and development planning;
- 7.3.2 design and development inputs;
- 7.3.3 design and development outputs;
- 7.3.4 design and development review;
- 7.3.5 design and development verification.

Note that up to and including clause 7.3.5, no manufacturing has taken place and/or no service has been provided.

Design and development validation (ISO 9001, clause 7.3.6)

The design and development clause 7.3.6 certainly has to be discussed during the first five stages of a design (clauses 7.3.1 to 7.3.5). The purpose of clause 7.3.6 is to forge agreement on how the proposed product or service is to be checked to the mutual satisfaction of the customer and the manufacturer/provider, before such activities begin.

In certain circumstances, there may be difficulties in deciding how validation of a product or provision of a service is to be carried out, but there are usually ways to resolve such problems to the satisfaction of both parties. For instance, a manufacturer of a high-technology printed circuit board cannot always carry out a full validation at the manufacturer's premises, because the manufacturer is unlikely to have the equipment into which the board is to be placed. However, the manufacturer might agree to provide, for example, five such completed circuit boards for placing inside the customer's machines, on other sites, to determine whether they are satisfactory. If they are, further production can go ahead without any changes.

It is inevitable, especially with large and complex products, that during the design and development stages some changes might be requested by the customer and some might be requested by the manufacturer of a product or the provider of a service. It is very important that any such requests for changes should be fully documented and, if any changes are agreed, both parties sign to that effect.

Manufacturing companies

Some exclusions from clause 7 are easy to justify and these have been referred to in Chapter 7. However, exclusion of the design and development clause is not always so simple, as exemplified by the cases given below.

Clause 7.3 is unlikely to cause any problems for some manufacturers. For instance, if a manufacturer merely manufactures a product to a third-party specification, be it the customer's own specification or some other specification acceptable to the customer, then the manufacturer can justifiably claim that clause 7.3 can be excluded as far as product made to that specification is concerned. The same is true for any products made by any company for customers in accordance with clearly defined and mutually acceptable third-party specifications.

However, what is the position if a company, which has justifiably excluded clause 7.3, then decides after manufacturing the first batch of a product that the product can be improved? Alternatively, a customer might suggest to the manufacturer that the product would be even more acceptable if certain changes could be made to the design before the next batch is produced.

If it is agreed that the manufacturer should make changes to the original specification, the manufacturer is in fact undertaking development work to improve the original design. The range of possible development work might extend from being a relatively trivial change to a much bigger change in the specification. Would the earlier justified exclusion of clause 7.3 now become unjustifiable? The author thinks not. Moreover, if a trivial change means that clause 7.3 can be excluded, at what point does a trivial change become non-trivial to the extent that clause 7.3 can no longer be excluded? Auditors should refer such difficulties to their accredited certification bodies in order to get a definitive answer to such problems.

(Incidentally, it has been assumed that the manufacturer has not been presented with a new updated specification for the next production batch. If this were the case, the manufacturer would not as a result be involved with design or development work, only perhaps with re-tooling, etc. so that the original justified exclusion would still apply as far as the task in question is concerned.)

Since the scenario given above is not the exception, but rather more commonplace, this does mean that many manufacturing companies will not be able to exclude clause 7.3, as was the case under the 1994 standard, by seeking certification to ISO 9002:1994 rather than ISO 9001:1994.

Service organizations

Consider a service industry that does not manufacture any products, but merely provides services. A field marketing company is one such case. A typical field marketing company will have many clients and its core business is providing appropriate field marketing personnel, on a short-term or long-term basis for their clients over a wide range of marketing opportunities.

The selected field marketing personnel might operate as sales teams, undertake merchandising, provide road shows, give demonstrations, undertake auditing in the marketplace, or carry out 'mystery shopping'.

In practice, the following sequence of events occurs. The company's client presents its needs and expectations. These are carefully examined. The field marketing company prepares a detailed cost proposal, which if successful is checked and re-checked before the operational stage. Whatever the proposed operational activities, they are based on previous experience over a number of years so that the company has a more-or-less standard approach for implementing the activities such as those listed above. There may be some fine-tuning of a proposed activity in order to satisfy the different needs of clients. Fine-tuning will, in any case, take place from time to time based on the company's earlier experience with similar activities, with the same client or with other clients.

Are the proposals for such service activities to be considered as design work and is the fine-tuning to be considered as development work? The author thinks neither is the case, but there may be exceptions to the general rule. Again, auditors are advised to refer borderline cases to their certification bodies.

Hospitals

Can clause 7.3 be justifiably excluded from a quality manual system for a hospital that is seeking ISO 9001 certification? In order to decide this, each clause of 7.3 is examined below against the processes that all patients take when they go to a hospital for diagnosis and treatment (see process diagrams PD 101–PD 105).

Design and development planning (ISO 9001, clause 7.3.1)

This clause will be addressed after clause 7.3.7. If other clauses, or most of them, cannot be addressed, then this clause too becomes irrelevant.

Design and development inputs (ISO 9001, clause 7.3.2)

When a patient is admitted to a hospital, after being taken through standard admission procedures the patient is made as comfortable as possible as quickly as possible. Shortly thereafter, an assessment is made by a professional person, such as a consultant in medicine, a consultant surgeon, a consultant psychiatrist, or a nurse therapist (hereafter referred to as a professional) to determine how to achieve the best possible quality of life for the patient. Once the initial and preliminary diagnosis is complete, it is usual to record the findings in the patient's case notes in a few simple explicit notes summarizing the general state of the patient and making clear what is to be done for the benefit of the patient. Such notes might be amended by the professional when the results of certain tests and investigations have been carried out.

Functional and performance requirements [ISO 9001, clause 7.3.2(a)]

In overall terms, the requirement for all patients is to improve their quality of life. The functional and performance input requirements are in fact derived from the initial diagnosis, but they might become even more specific as the diagnosis progresses to completion. In many cases, the diagnosis of the cause of the symptoms might be clear cut. For example, if third degree heart-block is diagnosed, the required input is treatment that will return cardiac rhythm to something like normal, by implantation of a cardiac pacemaker.

Applicable statutory and regulatory requirements [ISO 9001, clause 7.3.2(b)]

It is axiomatic that a professional person responsible for patient care will abide by any statutory and regulatory requirements.

Information derived from previous similar designs [ISO 9001, clause 7.3.2(c)]

All professionals in charge of patient care will automatically draw on their knowledge and experience.

Other requirements essential for design and development [ISO 9001, clause 7.3.2(d)]

There are no requirements other than those specified above. If there were, the professional would not have done their job properly.

It would appear that the whole of clause 7.3.2, design and development inputs, can be addressed.

Design and development outputs (ISO 9001, clause 7.3.3)

Meeting the input requirements [ISO 9001, clause 7.3.3(a)]

In the case of a patient in third degree heart-block, the proposed output required is the implantation of a cardiac pacemaker. Many patients have benefited from such implants world-wide. The quality of life for the vast majority of patients is restored to normal, with a very high degree of confidence by the cardiologist and the surgeon, after relatively minor surgery.

In other surgical cases, however, the outcome might be less certain. In cases of cancer, before a patient undergoes surgery they will normally have undergone other processes beforehand, e.g. a radiological examination to provide the maximum amount of diagnostic information possible for the surgeon. Other supplementary processes may include the sterilization of surgical tools, anaesthesia and electrocardiography readings. In spite of all such back-up, the expected output from surgery cannot always be defined with certainty beforehand. Moreover, the diagnoses, even using modern technology, do not always reveal beforehand the full extent of the problem in a given patient. Thus the output cannot be defined with a high degree of certainty before surgery, but only after surgical intervention (and perhaps not even then). Thus, there is no question of being able to compare design and development input, i.e. the need to achieve an improved quality of life of a patient, with design and development output before surgery commences.

With other diagnoses that do not involve surgery, the outcome of any proposed treatment might also be less certain. In such cases outputs can be established only, and therefore recorded only, after medical intervention. Thus, again there is no question of being able to compare design and development input, i.e. the need to achieve an improved quality of life of a patient, with design and development output before treatment has taken place.

Clause 7.3.3(a) cannot be addressed with certainty before action is taken, so clause 7.3.3(a) can therefore be justifiably excluded.

Provide appropriate information for purchasing, production and for service provisions [ISO 9001, clause 7.3.3(b)]

Any requirements for use by the professionals in connection with routine diagnoses and therapies, e.g. pacemakers, drugs and equipment, will have been addressed through the usual channels by requests to management, pharmacy, estates or purchasing.

Clause 7.3.3(b) can be addressed.

Contain or reference product acceptance criteria [ISO 9001, clause 7.3.3(c)]

As explained earlier in this chapter, design and development outputs should include or make reference to specific acceptance criteria before manufacture commences or before the provision of a service begins.

All professionals in hospitals strive to improve the quality of lives of their patients. They cannot define specific acceptance criteria before treatment commences because medicine and surgery are not exact sciences. In reality, any improved quality of life of the patient might have to be acceptable, but this cannot be known with certainty for a patient before treatment commences.

Clause 7.3(c) is about agreeing acceptance criteria for checking that a customer or a patient gets what they want, what they ordered, what the specification or contract states and, moreover, getting precisely what has been agreed before manufacture or the provision of a service. In the treatment of patients there is no such certainty before treatment begins.

Clause 7.3.3(c) cannot be addressed.

Specify the characteristics of the product that are essential for its safe and proper use [ISO 9001, clause 7.3.3(d)]

In the field of manufacturing, this clause means that, for instance, an electric kettle must be electrically safe to use when used in the way for which it was designed, namely to boil water. In the case of a patient in a hospital, the product is the improved quality of life of the patient, but this cannot be defined precisely before treatment commences.

Clause 7.3.3(d) cannot be addressed.

Design and development review (ISO 9001, clause 7.3.4)

In a hospital there is no final design and development review about what is going to be done, before anything is done so as to ensure that the output will match the input. The professionals are well aware that they cannot be certain that the actual output (as opposed to the designed output) will indeed match the input. This is precisely what this clause is about. In practice, professionals in a hospital decide what they are going to do and do it or ensure that it is done.

Clause 7.3.4 cannot be addressed because reviews do not usually take place before treatment.

Design and development verification (ISO 9001, clause 7.3.5)

The final clause that has to be addressed in any design and development work is for the design to be verified, ideally by a person (or persons) not previously associated with it, to ensure that the design does in fact satisfy the input requirements.

In a hospital such work leading to an improved quality of life of patients has been done by other bodies. Thus, it is not the job of a professional in a hospital to explain how the proposed service (medical treatment or surgery) will be verified before implementation of medical treatment or surgery. Since the thalidomide scandal in the early 1960s, most governments now require by law properly organized clinical trials to validate drugs before they become generally available to ensure that they are safe and are likely to achieve what is expected of them. The Medicines Control Agency is the regulatory body in the UK. Likewise, implants such as cardiac pacemakers have to be approved by regulatory bodies before they can be generally used by professionals. In a hospital, once a professional has decided what needs to be done, treatment is carried out and hopefully it improves the quality of life of the patient.

If there is little or no response to treatment the professional has to reconsider the method of treatment.

Clause 7.3.5, the verification clause, is not applicable. Professionals are not required to refer their proposed therapy to other professionals for verification.

Design and development validation (ISO 9001, clause 7.3.6)

Before manufacture of a product or provision of a service, there is a requirement for both parties to agree on how the actual output will be verified to ensure that the agreed designed output does in fact agree with the designed input.

The designed output for a hospital patient is an improved quality of life for a patient. This cannot be guaranteed and also the degree of an improved quality of life for a patient may be, at least partially, a subjective matter.

Clause 7.3.6 cannot be addressed.

Control of design and development changes (ISO 9001, clause 7.3.7)

In a hospital the treatment might have to be changed from time to time as the state of a patient changes, or if a patient does not respond as expected to the chosen treatment. Similarly, in the case of surgery, a proposed surgical procedure might have to be changed during an operation as new evidence presents itself, which necessitates a change in the planned surgery. In either of these cases, a professional is in complete control and can change the treatment or surgery as deemed necessary without reference to anyone else.

Clause 7.3.7 cannot be addressed. Professionals are not required to refer their proposed changes in treatment to other professionals

Design and development planning (ISO 9001, clause 7.3.1)

Since only the input clause (7.3.2) and purchasing clause [7.3.3 (b)] can be addressed, clause 7.3.1 becomes irrelevant.

Summary

It would appear that only the input clause and the purchasing clause can be addressed when dealing with patients in hospitals. All the other clauses cannot be addressed, either because the output cannot be certain before treatment occurs, or because they are not applicable because of the way in which professionals have clinical freedom (within certain limitations, such as evidence-based medicine) on how they treat their patients.

The purpose of clause 7.3 is to ensure that there is a very high degree of certainty that the customer will get precisely what has been agreed before manufacturing begins or before the provision of a service commences. Even when such certainties do exist in patient treatment, the clinical freedom granted to professionals precludes the actions required by the other clauses. In such circumstances, the whole of clause 7.3 on design and development can be justifiably excluded from the quality manual.

Chapter 10: Clinical audits

Clinical audit endeavours to improve patient care and patient outcomes by systematically reviewing care against explicit criteria. The Commission for Health Improvement (CHI) in 2000, and later the Commission for Healthcare Audit and Inspection (CHAI) in 2004 (see Appendix 3) acquired overall responsibility for developing clinical audit programmes for England and Wales. Clinical audit is now included in clinical governance reviews. Some of the earlier clinical audits were not satisfactory in that, for instance, national standards where they existed were not always used as a reference. Because of such shortcomings an Office for Information on Healthcare Performance (OIHP) was established. Its terms of reference are to:

- promote first-class clinical audits as an essential element of a wider performance assessment framework;
- ensure that the first-class clinical audits are linked with other aspects of CHAI's work (e.g. clinical governance reviews);
- endeavour to improve patient care and patient outcomes as a result of clinical audits.

Some of the ongoing national clinical audits include:

- myocardial infarction national audit project (MINAP);
- venus ulcers;
- violence in mental health settings;
- stroke.

Other national clinical audits that are planned for are:

- lung cancer;
- head and neck cancers;
- evidenced-based recommendations for the elderly;
- breast cancer;
- colorectal cancer; and
- diabetes.

CHAI will now endorse only clinical audits that satisfy its own criteria. The criteria for endorsing clinical audits are still being developed and it is hoped that, as a result, the standard of clinical audits will be improved in all hospitals. The criteria will be based on the best aspects of clinical audits developed locally and on those that have been developed nationally.

The fundamental aim of all clinical audits is to improve patient care and patient outcomes. Hence one criterion for endorsing future clinical audits will be the involvement of patients, particularly at steering group level. Effective involvement of patients and the public in running clinical audits should ensure that clinical audits reflect the needs of patients and, hopefully, this will result in improvements in patient care and patient outcomes.

Clinical audit schedule: selection of processes to be audited

Until recently, a hospital could decide for itself which activities should be audited. Hitherto, this could be decided by a chief executive, a medical director or by a director of nursing, or a committee that is likely to include one of more of the aforementioned senior members of staff. This state of affairs is to change. In future, CHAI will insist that all clinical audits will have to meet its own criteria including patient involvement.

A good starting point for any discussions on a schedule for clinical audits is the general patient process for all patients, as depicted in process diagram, PD 101 (Chapter 3). Other process diagrams such as PD 102 to 105 depict the major processes that take place in different departments. It might be agreed that all of the major hospital processes ought to undergo clinical audit first and this should be noted on the audit schedule. These could then become the basis of a second round of more detailed departmental clinical audits either in the immediate future or in the ensuing year depending on the outcomes of the first round of clinical audits. During the more detailed departmental clinical audits an auditor would be expected to refer to any relevant hospital protocols, procedures and policies in connection with the diagnosis, treatment and care of patients. There will also be the reports issued, for instance, by the hospital's risk management committee that might be particularly relevant to a certain audit. The clinical audit schedule will also be influenced by the national audits referred to earlier. In addition, any of the reports issued by NICE, NSF and NPSA (Appendix 3) that are relevant to a particular department must not be ignored. Reports from professional bodies such as the royal colleges might also have a bearing on some aspects of the clinical audits undertaken by a hospital. All such relevant internal documents and external documents, as they are sometimes referred to in connection with the international quality management systems standard, should be systematically considered when the clinical audit schedule and associated audit planning are taking place.

It is strongly recommended that all members of staff are also invited to suggest areas that might benefit from clinical audits, since some may well be more aware than senior staff about the problems that arise in patient care despite the process diagrams, etc.

Other areas that need to be audited might arise from information received from patients, carers and other organizations devoted to the interests of patients. Such information might also arise from patient satisfaction surveys, similar to the monitoring of customer satisfaction surveys that are mandatory in ISO 9001 work.

Patient complaints need not be addressed directly by clinical audit since the Patient Advisory and Liaison Service (PALS) now deals with patient complaints and this service will be reviewed separately by CHAI under the general remit of clinical governance. Nevertheless, patients might make their views known and others may be asked for their views.

Once a list has been made, it will inevitably be necessary to give priorities to some audits over others and such considerations will determine the clinical audit schedule. Once a clinical audit schedule has been agreed and approved by top management, it should not be possible to change it without the approval of the chief executive.

There are no such choices with ISO 9001. Some audits will be given priority over others, but internal auditing must cover the whole of an organization's activities that fall within the scope of the certificate being sought by an organization or that has been awarded to an organization.

The four stages of a clinical audit

When clinical auditing begins, the first objective is to establish that the existing planned arrangements are being followed by clinicians (and other hospital staff). In other words the auditors must decide from the objective evidence collected whether the current clinical practice conforms to the planned arrangements that aim to improve patient care and patient outcomes.

The second stage is to consider whether changes ought to be made to improve the current clinical practice for the benefit of patients.

Thirdly, an audit must determine whether any changes made, for whatever reasons, are indeed beneficial to patients.

Finally, at each stage of the clinical audit, the views of patients and the public are paramount:

- at the steering group stage;
- at the planning stage of an audit;
- during execution of the planned stage;
- when considering changes that are intended to be beneficial to patients;
- when checking that the actual changes really are beneficial to patients.

Attributes of good clinical auditors

Clinical auditors need to have the appropriate personality be able to ask searching questions of people with diverse personalities and be able to cope with people who consider themselves to be very important in the hospital set-up. These people may feel that they really ought not to be questioned because of their standing. Such people need to be handled politely, but firmly, with a quiet determination on the part of the auditor to obtain the objective evidence that is required. It should have been made clear by top management that nobody, including themselves, can be exempt from questioning by auditors. The author's experience is that the vast majority of people do not object to being questioned by an experienced auditor. Those that do usually have something to hide. Even in such circumstances an indefatigable auditor will quietly and politely rise to the challenge and eventually get the objective evidence that is required.

Clinical auditors are strongly recommended to seek training in auditing. Auditors who conduct auditing on behalf of certification bodies are required to undergo rigorous training and monitoring before they are allowed to undertake audits on behalf of accredited certification bodies. The same should be true of clinical auditors. With ISO 9001, no auditor is allowed to audit their own work. This should also be the case with clinical audits. It is the view of the author that any good auditor can audit any activity, including those in hospitals. They can also conduct clinical audits, although knowledge of hospitals does make it easier.

Clinical audits and ISO 9001 auditing

Clinical audits in hospitals differ in some respects from internal auditing conducted in other organizations based on ISO 9001 (see clause 8.2.2 and PC 103), but there are many similarities. A few of the similarities are given below.

- Clinical audits should begin on the scheduled date. The lead auditor should be in charge of an audit, although several auditors might be required to carry out the audit. The lead auditor must chair the opening meeting. Who else attends can be decided by the head of the department. The opening meeting can be brief, usually not more than about half an hour. The chair will remind those present which activities are to be audited. They will also stress what clinical auditing is all about, i.e. what the overall objectives are. A tentative plan of action is usually preferred so that people in a large department know approximately when auditors are likely to visit different areas of the department. Randomly selected patients will be interviewed and some patient records will be examined. A tentative time is set for a closing meeting at which the findings will be summarized.
- Patient confidentiality will, of course, be maintained at all times in accordance with the hospital's guideline document on this matter.
- The findings of clinical audits must be viewed in a positive manner, because they afford opportunities to hospital departments and probably for the entire hospital to consider ways of improving the care of patients.
- Audits must focus on objective evidence. During an actual audit opinions and hearsay are irrelevant. They might well be relevant after the findings of an audit have been recorded but certainly not before.
- Whenever auditors find that there is a deviation from the planned patient routes, as specified in the relevant process diagrams, a nonconformity should be recorded on a prescribed form. The recorded nonconformity is the basis for future discussions with all concerned. This might include clinicians, other staff, perhaps the medical director, the nursing director and the chief executive. The agreed corrective action(s) must be recorded and followed through to completion. Verification that the corrective action has been carried out has to be confirmed before the audit can be completed satisfactorily.
- All auditors should be aware of all the internal and external documents that are relevant to a given audit. If the contents of such documents are being ignored by hospital staff, in part or in their entirety, nonconformities need to be raised and recorded as explained in the previous section.
- Any discerning auditor might discover an untoward event (an adverse event or a near-miss event). These should have been reported to top management on discovery. A good auditor will record such an occurrence either as a nonconformity, if it has just been discovered, or as an observation, if it has been reported already. Whatever is the case, the auditor should check that appropriate corrective action has taken place to prevent reoccurrence.

- Similarly, an auditor might become aware of an apparent unnecessary risk to a patient that has not been realized hitherto. This should be recorded as an observation for the benefit of the department being audited and, perhaps more importantly, for the hospital's risk management committee.
- Patient complaints are similarly not within the explicit remit of clinical audits since it is now mandatory for every hospital to have a process in place for dealing with patient complaints (Appendix 3). If coincidentally, an auditor receives a complaint from a patient, an observation should be recorded to check that action has or is being taken.
- Records on all clinical audits must be maintained for study and review by an appropriate committee that must include top management. This is no different from what happens with ISO 9001 internal audits in which such reports are discussed at the management review meetings.
- CHAI will examine all clinical audits as part of their clinical governance inspections. In the same way, external auditors from ISO 9001 certification bodies always examine the internal audits of organizations seeking certification to the international standard.
- An examination of a typical patient process from referral by a general practitioner to the time of discharge from a hospital (see Chapter 3, PD 107) provides an indication of the amount of data that might be collected about a patient experience and on hospital activities that have a bearing on the patient experience. A lot of information and data about diagnosis and treatment are usually collected. Some are collated and analysed. Data about timings are also relevant to the patient experience and should be collected, collated and analysed. A patient is concerned about the time between stage 1 and stage 11, whereas government waiting times focus on the time between stage 8 and stage 11. Top management should be focusing on all these aspects so that continual improvements can be made in the ways in which the hospital functions so that patients receive the best possible care and outcomes from every point of view.

Clinical auditing and an ISO 9001 certificate

There is one important difference between clinical auditing in a hospital and ISO 9001 internal auditing in other types of organization. If internal auditing conducted under the aegis of ISO 9001 indicates all of the criteria required for the award of an ISO 9001 certificate have been met, then an external audit by a well trained and experienced auditor, conducted on behalf of an accredited certification body, is likely to confirm that this is the case and an ISO 9001 certificate is likely to be awarded.

In the case of clinical audit in a hospital, however good the findings, it will not necessarily result in the award of an ISO 9001 certificate, since all the criteria for the ISO 9001 certificate are unlikely to have been addressed unless other specific steps have been taken to address all the requirements of the standard. Thus, the award of an ISO 9001 certificate by an independent accredited certification body can be looked upon as a further step, in addition to clinical audit, towards achieving quality patient care throughout an entire hospital.

Chapter 11: Guideline audit questions

Introduction

These guideline audit questions can be used by hospital staff when they undertake internal audits. The first part of the chapter focuses on the requirements of ISO 9001. The second part addresses the requirements of clinical audits. Many of the aspects of ISO 9001 auditing also apply to clinical auditing (see Chapter 10). As with ISO 9001 auditing, regulatory and statutory requirements must also be addressed in clinical auditing. However, with clinical audits additional cognizance must also be taken by clinicians in response to the recommendations and requirements of publications issued by other national organizations such as NICE and NSF (see Appendix 3).

ISO 9001 audits

As explained in the previous chapters the revised standard focuses on the processes by which a hospital meets the needs and expectations of patients by attempting to achieve an improved quality of life for patients, where possible.

Every hospital should have several overall major process such as PD 101, PD 105 and PD 106. There are many other departmental major processes, such as PD 102, PD 103 and PD 104. Each major process proceeds to completion through planned sequential steps supported by one or more lower-level processes and, sometimes, with notes attached to the stages within a process document (see Chapter 3).

In view of this new focus on processes, the new emphasis in auditing is on process auditing. Process auditing means that the auditor is checking the sequential and interrelated steps from the beginning of a major process of planned activities until the patient in question is discharged from hospital. The interrelated steps might be the processes in other departments, such as lower-level processes, the notes within a process diagram as well as other referenced documents. Such auditing, known as process auditing, might prove to be more attractive and understandable to some, because they relate more easily to the purpose of auditing that now focuses on patient experiences in hospitals and patient outcomes.

In spite of this new emphasis on process auditing, there will still be a need for some compliance auditing. Compliance auditing will be necessary when checking on the stand-alone processes, such as sterilization of surgical instruments, confirming that the relevant requirements of the standard have been addressed.

It is clearly impossible to produce an all-embracing list of audit questions for universal major processes. However, it is possible to compile a comprehensive list of typical audit questions that address the requirements of ISO 9001. The reader, when process auditing, can select the relevant questions when following a specific audit trail through a major process pausing, as necessary, when interacting processes intervene until the intended output is achieved. Compliance auditing is much more straightforward and likely to be less time consuming, but the specific questions listed should also be of help to those conducting this type of audit.

Another approach to be recommended to inexperienced auditors is to concentrate on particular clauses of the standard. Concentration on a particular clause is recommended until the requirements are understood and ideas on how to address them can be written down. Usually, there are different approaches that can be taken to ascertain whether requirements have been addressed. Other auditors can be asked how they would decide on suitable questions to find out how requirements have been met. This will lead to the auditor becoming fully familiar with the requirements of the standard, knowing how to address them and, after carrying out one or two process audits or compliance audits that involve the clauses in question, only occasionally will it be necessary to refer to the relevant audit questions in this chapter. If auditing decisions are ever challenged, the auditor will then be in a strong position to answer any criticisms.

Chapter 10 outlines the atributes of a good clinical auditor. Auditing is not just about having a list of possible questions. Newcomers to auditing might benefit from reading *ISO 9000 Quality Systems Auditing* [8].

Clinical audits

As already explained (see Chapter 10 and Appendix 3) the Commission for Healthcare Audit and Improvements (CHAI) is now responsible for reviewing clinical audits as part of its hospital inspection process under clinical governance.

Any clinical audit has four main aspects. Is the patient process in accordance with what has been planned and agreed? Are the patient outcomes satisfactory? Have the needs and expectations of patients been satisfied? Is appropriate data being collected, collated and analysed for the hospital and, when considered necessary, for comparison with national data?

Quality management system (ISO 9001, clause 4)

General requirements (ISO 9001, clause 4.1)

I understand that you have established a quality management system.
Has it been fully implemented?
How is it maintained?

What do you understand by the requirement that the hospital must continually improve the effectiveness of your quality management system?

Please explain the major processes of the hospital.
Can you show me examples of such processes in connection with:

- management activities?
- provision of resources?
- diagnosis and treatment of patients?
- other services in connection with patient care?
- monitoring and measurements on patients?
- monitoring and measurements indirectly related to patient care, e.g.sterilization of instruments?

Do you use lower-level processes? Can you please show me examples?

Please show me how the lower-level processes interrelate with the major processes at the appropriate times and that they all function as planned.

What criteria and methods are used to ensure that the operation and control of major and lower-level processes are effective?

How do you ensure the availability of appropriate resources?

How do you ensure that appropriate documentation/information is always readily available to support the operation and monitoring of the processes?

What monitoring and measurements take place during the processes, followed by analyses, to ensure that planned results are achieved?

Have such monitoring, measurements and analyses ever resulted in continual improvements being made in the processes?
Can you please give me examples?

Are any processes that could affect clinical outputs outsourced, i.e. the planned improvement in the quality of life of patients?
Are any processes outsourced such as those provided for other staff that are responsible for services in connection with patient care?
Are outsourced processes clearly identified in the quality management system?
How are outsourced processes controlled?
Please can I see examples of controlled outsourcing?

Documentation requirements (ISO 9001, clause 4.2)

General (ISO 9001, clause 4.2.1)

Can you show me the documentation on which the quality management system is based?
Is it partly or wholly on your intranet site?
If it is on your intranet, who has the read/write facility?

How many hard copies of the quality manual are there?
Can I please see some copies?
Are they uniquely identified?
What are their issue numbers?
What are the dates on the quality manual?

Can I please see your quality policy statement?
How many have been issued?

Are the quality policy documents controlled documents?

Can I please see a list of your quality objectives?
These might be changed from time to time.
How are changes controlled and disseminated?

Please may I see the mandatory procedures:

- control of documents?
- control of records?
- internal audit?
- control of nonconforming product?
- corrective action?
- preventive action?

These will be examined in detail at appropriate times during an audit.

Please show me any other documentation (process diagrams, procedures, policies, work instructions and forms) that are necessary for control of the quality management system.

Please show me any other documentation (protocols, procedures, flow diagrams, work instructions, forms and internal documents) that is being used by the hospital to ensure effective planning, operation and control of all the major and lower-level processes.

Are notes attached to any of the stages in the processes?

Am I correct in saying that you have established records that provide objective evidence of conformity to requirements and the effective operation of your quality management system?

Do you have a comprehensive list of such records?

Can I sample a number of these records now please?
(I will ask to see other records as and when deemed appropriate.)

Quality manual (ISO 9001, clause 4.2.2)

Does the quality manual include the scope of the quality management system?
Please may I see it?

Have all requirements of the standard been addressed?
If not, are the exclusions from clause 7 recorded in the quality manual?
Have you justified in the quality manual the reasons for the exclusions?
Please will you go through the arguments for such exclusions now?

Does the quality manual include a description of the sequence and interaction of all the major processes?
Please show me how you have achieved this.

Does the quality manual make reference to procedures at appropriate points in the text?
Please show me examples.
Does the quality manual include procedures or are they compiled separately?
If procedures are filed separately from the quality manual are the procedures listed in the quality manual?

Control of documents (ISO 9001, clause 4.2.3)

The control of documents procedure must explain how the quality management system documents are controlled. The procedure, together with the quality manual, must answer the following questions.

Who finally approves documents (the quality manual, process diagrams, procedures, protocols, work instructions and forms) for adequacy, before they are allowed to become part of the quality management system?
Please show me evidence of this.

How are documents identifiable?
Do they have unique reference letters and/or numbers?
How does the hospital ensure that all documents are readily available?
How does the hospital ensure that all documents remain legible?

What arrangements are in place for reviewing, updating, and reapproving such documents prior to reissue?

How is the revision status of a document, or part of a document, identified?
Please show me examples.
How are changes in a document identified?
Please show me examples.

How does the management representative, or another named person, ensure that relevant versions of applicable documents are always available at points of use or application?
Please show me an example.

How are documents of external origin (e.g. standards, codes of practice and forms) controlled to ensure that only the latest issues of such documents can be used?
Is there a master list of external documents?

What happens to superseded documents?
What precautions are taken to prevent unintended use of obsolete documents?
Are the superseded documents returned to the management representative, or another person, on receipt of an updated document or when a document is no longer applicable?
Is one copy, clearly marked 'superseded', filed separately, and retained for knowledge preservation purposes?

Is the quality policy statement a controlled document?
How is the quality policy statement document controlled?
Does it have a unique number and issue number?

Is the statement of quality objectives a controlled document?
How do you control the quality objectives document?

Control of records (ISO 9001, clause 4.2.4)

What is the purpose of keeping records?

The control of records procedure must explain how the quality management system records are controlled. The procedure, together with the quality manual, must answer the following questions.

Does it include a list of records that have to be kept for purposes of ISO 9001:2000?

Are records always clearly identifiable?
Please show me examples.

Are all records stored carefully?
Can I please see how they are stored?

Can all records be retrieved easily?
How, for instance, can I retrieve *x document*?

Are all records protected from possible damage?
Show me examples of protection.

Are all records legible and do they remain legible?
Please can I see some of your older records?

Have retention times of different records been defined?
Please give examples and explain any different requirements.

Are any patient records kept on microfiche?
At what stage is this done?
Can I please see examples?
Who is responsible for the microfiche of patient records?
Is there a procedure on the microfiche of patient records?

Who has the authority to dispose of records?
Can you give me an example of disposal and the authority for such disposal?

Management responsibility (ISO 9001, clause 5)

Management commitment (ISO 9001, clause 5.1)

These comments are addressed to a member of top management (e.g. the chief executive or managing director).

I have already spent some time seeking objective evidence about your quality management system based on ISO 9001. I am impressed (or unimpressed) by what I have found so far during the audit. Everyone has been most courteous and helpful (or courteous, but reluctantly helpful, or whatever is appropriate).
Would you kindly let them know what I feel?

The revised standard makes it clear that top management has to be actively involved in the hospital's quality management system. All requirements in clause 5 begin: 'Top management shall... '.

I have asked to spend a little time with you because I hope you will be able to convince me of your commitment to the development and implementation of your quality management system and your commitment to continual improvement in the effectiveness of your hospital's quality management system. With these points in mind, I would like to ask you a few questions.

I have read your quality policy, signed by you, and dated...

What do you think about having to provide a quality policy statement for your hospital?

What are your views on having to establish quality objectives?

Do you chair the management review meetings?
Are they particularly enlightening from a management point of view?

Who is responsible for ensuring that adequate resources are available for the development, implementation and continual improvement of the quality management system?

How do you ensure that all employees are aware of striving at all times to improve the quality of life of all patients?

At the end of the interview an auditor must make a judgement as to whether top management is committed to the development, implementation and continual improvement in the effectiveness of the quality management system. The final judgement will be influenced to some extent by any objective evidence obtained earlier and later in the audit, hence the importance of not interviewing top management at the beginning of an audit.

There are four possibilities for subjective and objective evidence.

Subjective evidence and objective evidence good

If the somewhat subjective evidence collected arising from the discussion with top management is good and the objective evidence collected earlier was good, then the commitment of top management to the quality management system would appear to be satisfactory.

Subjective evidence good and objective evidence poor

If the subjective evidence is good, but the objective evidence collected earlier was poor, then top management has evidently failed to develop and implement its quality management system satisfactorily.

Subjective evidence bad/poor and objective evidence good

If the subjective evidence is bad, or poor, and the objective evidence collected earlier was good, this would suggest the quality management system is functioning satisfactory in spite of the lack of enthusiastic commitment of top management.

Subjective evidence bad/poor and objective evidence poor

If the subjective evidence is bad or poor and the objective evidence collected earlier was poor, then it can be safely assumed that the quality management system is operating under most unsatisfactory conditions with little commitment of top management.

In both of the circumstances in which the subjective evidence is suggesting lack of top management commitment, an auditor would be wise to refrain from commenting until the closing meeting of the audit. By that time the auditor might have collected other damaging objective evidence to support earlier impressions of the lack of commitment of top management.

Customer focus (ISO 9001, clause 5.2)

One of the requirements in the standard is to ensure that the needs and expectations of patients are determined and are then converted into patient requirements so that through the hospital's major processes it is evident that the hospital is striving at all times to improve the quality of life of all patients.

It is axiomatic that clinical staff strive at all times to improve the quality of life of patients.

How does the hospital address other patient needs, such as:

- privacy?
- common courtesies?
- cleanliness at all times and in all places?
- good food?

What else does the hospital do to ensure that the needs and expectations of patients are addressed?

Are patient processes, or process diagrams, planned in such a way that patients attending the hospital for diagnosis or therapy are routinely dealt with in an expeditious manner (excluding emergencies)?

Quality policy (ISO 9001, clause 5.3)

I have read carefully your quality policy statement signed by you (or whomever) and dated...
It seems appropriate for your kind of hospital and is positive in every respect.

How do you ensure that people at all levels in your hospital know about the quality policy and understand what it means?

How do you ensure that the quality policy is reviewed for its continuing suitability?

I note the commitment of top management to comply with the requirements of ISO 9001. Can you give me one or more examples in which the requirements of the standard have resulted in changes in the ways in which the hospital functions?

I note your commitment continually to improve the effectiveness of the quality management system.
What do you understand by this statement?
How do you go about ensuring that this happens?

Planning (ISO 9001, clause 5.4)

Quality objectives (ISO 9001, clause 5.4.1)

How does the hospital decide on measurable quality objectives?
Are they set for higher levels of management/senior staff as well as for junior staff or at department level?

Is there a framework for establishing and reviewing quality objectives in a systematic manner?
Please explain and show me examples.

Are all of the quality objectives compatible with the quality policy statement?

Quality management system planning (ISO 9001, clause 5.4.2)

When planning the quality management system were the general requirements of the quality management system addressed (see clause 4.1) as well as the quality objectives (see clause 5.4.1)?

When changes to the quality management system are planned and implemented, who is responsible for ensuring that the integrity of the quality management system is maintained?

Can you please show me an example of such a change?

Responsibility, authority and communication (ISO 9001, clause 5.5)

Responsibility and authority (ISO 9001, clause 5.5.1)

How do you ensure that responsibilities and authorities are defined and communicated within the hospital?

Does the hospital have an organization chart?
Please may I see it?

If the organization chart is not in general circulation, how are employees expected to know who is responsible for what?

If there are no names, or very few names, on the hospital chart, how do individuals know who reports to whom?

Are the responsibilities and authorities of individuals clearly specified?
Please show me examples.

Management representative (ISO 9001, clause 5.5.2)

Has management appointed a management representative (or quality manager)?

Have their responsibilities been defined?
Where is this documented?

How does management ensure that the responsibilities and authority of the management representative for establishing, implementing and maintaining the quality management system is known to all members of staff?

What measures have been taken to ensure that staff are aware that the management representative has a direct line of responsibility to you?
May I please see your latest hospital organization chart again?

To whom does the management representative report on the performance of the quality management system?
Please show me examples of such reporting.

To whom does the management representative report on the need for any changes to improve the quality management system?
Can you show me such examples?

How does the management representative ensure the promotion of awareness of patient requirements throughout the hospital?
Can you please show me examples of how such desirable requirements are promoted?

What other responsibilities, if any, does your management representative have?

Is the management representative responsible for liaison with external parties, e.g. certification bodies?
If not, who is responsible for such activities and what arrangements exist to ensure that the management representative is kept fully informed of such developments?

Internal communication (ISO 9001, clause 5.5.3)

How do you ensure that appropriate communication processes are established within your hospital?

How do you ensure that communication takes place within your hospital regarding the effectiveness of the quality management system?

Management review (ISO 9001, clause 5.6)

General (ISO 9001, clause 5.6.1)

What arrangements are in place for top management to review the quality management system to ensure its continuing suitability, adequacy and effectiveness?

What are the planned intervals between such meetings?
Please show me that the planned intervals between management review meetings have been kept.

Have the reviews of the quality management system shown that it continues to be suitable, adequate and effective for the hospital?

Have such reviews resulted in opportunities for changes to be made that have resulted in continual improvement in the effectiveness of the quality management system?
Please show me one example of such continual improvement.

The reviews provide opportunities for changes to be made to the quality policy. Have any such changes been made?

Have the reviews resulted in the need for changes to quality objectives?
Can you show me an example of such a change?

Are records kept of management review meetings (see clause 4.2.4)?
Please may I see the records of the last few management review meetings?

Review input (ISO 9001, clause 5.6.2)

Do you have a standard agenda for your management review meetings?

As a minimum, does it include the following:

(a) follow-up actions from earlier management reviews?

(b) the results of audits (both internal and any external audits)?

(c) improvements in patient processes?

(d) successes in achieving better quality of life for patients;

(e) failures to achieve improved quality of life for patients because of adverse events and near misses;

(f) status of corrective and preventive actions;

(g) patient feedback (patient complaints and answers to questionnaires on patient satisfaction);

(h) recommendations for improvement in the effectiveness of the quality management system;

(i) many changes, whatever their origin or nature, that could have a bearing on the quality management system?

Review output (ISO 9001, clause 5.6.3)

> Can you give me examples of decisions and actions decided at management review meetings that have resulted in:
>
> (a) improvement in the effectiveness of the quality management system and its processes;
>
> (b) improvements in the quality of life of patients;
>
> (c) the need for more resources?
>
> Do you have a standard agenda for a management review meeting?
> Please may I see one?

Resource management (ISO 9001, clause 6)

Provision of resources (ISO 9001, clause 6.1)

> Who is responsible for determining and providing resources needed for implementation and maintenance of the quality management system?
> Can I please see an example of this?
>
> What effort is given to determining and providing resources that will result in continual improvement in the effectiveness of the quality management system?
>
> Does the hospital determine and provide the resources needed to enhance patient satisfaction by:
>
> - helping clinicians to improve the quality of life of patients?
> - helping others to provide all the other services in connection with patient care?
>
> Please show me at least one example in each category

Human resources (ISO 9001, clause 6.2)

General (ISO 9001, clause 6.2.1)

> How do you ensure that clinical staff whose prime duties and responsibilities are to improve the quality of life of patients, and other staff who provide all the other services in connection with patient care, are competent for such tasks on the basis of their relevant education, training, skills and experience?
>
> Can you give me a few examples?

Competence, awareness and training (ISO 9001, clause 6.2.2)

Are competency needs defined for clinical staff who are responsible for achieving a better quality of life for patients and for all the other staff who are responsible for providing other services in connection with patient care?
Please show me several examples for clinicians and other staff.

How does the hospital arrange training, where necessary, or other actions to achieve the defined competences in those cases in which competency has been found wanting?
Can you please show me evidence of this?

How is in-house training (and any external training) evaluated?
Please can I see examples?

How do you ensure that all employees are made aware of the relevance and importance of their activities and how each one contributes in some way or other to the achievement of quality objectives?
How do you ensure that any new employees are suitably briefed on this matter?
Please show me examples.

How do you maintain appropriate records of all staff on education, training, skills and experience (see clause 4.2.4)?
Please may I choose, at random, some training records for examination?
Also, specifically, may I see the training record(s) of your internal auditor(s)?
How do you ensure that all records are kept up to date?

Infrastructure (ISO 9001, clause 6.3)

If a hospital is to continue to achieve an improved quality of life for patients, and ensure that other staff provide a satisfactory service in connection with patient care, then management has to determine, provide and maintain an appropriate infrastructure.

Who is responsible for providing and maintaining an appropriate infrastructure?

In particular, who is responsible for:

- buildings?
- wards?
- diagnostic and treatment areas?
- operating theatres?
- laboratories and associated facilities?
- the hospital's intranet and associated software?

Please show me examples.

How are decisions made on process requirements for major and lower-level processes?
Please give examples.
Who makes decisions on any support services that are necessary for clinicians who are striving to achieve an improved quality of life for patients?
Please give examples.

What support services are outsourced?
Who is responsible for ensuring that outsourced services are of the required standard?
Please show me examples.

Work environment (ISO 9001, clause 6.4)

How does management determine, provide and manage the human and physical factors of the work environment that are necessary for clinical staff to improve the quality of life of patients (as well as staff that provide other services in connection with patient care)?

Do these include:

- safety of individuals?
- ergonomics of working?
- appropriate lighting levels?
- appropriate temperature and humidity controls?
- acceptable noise levels?
- acceptable levels of cleanliness and hygiene?
- minimum pollution levels?
- appropriate protective equipment?

Which of the above are covered by legislation, regulations and codes of practice?

Does the hospital require special facilities, such as clean rooms and sterile areas?

How are such special requirements addressed?

What controls are in place to ensure that the planned work environments are maintained?

Product realization (ISO 9001, clause 7)

Planning of product realization (ISO 9001, clause 7.1)

Patient treatment plans will exist in many different forms, such as brief and simple plans for relatively simple diagnoses and treatment, or more detailed plans in the case of more complex diagnoses and treatment. It is axiomatic that any patient plan has one prime objective: to improve the quality of life of the patient. Non-clinical staff have the responsibility of ensuring that all the support services needed in connection with patient care are provided in a timely and efficient manner.

Can I please see several such quality plans?

Have all the processes been clearly identified (major processes, lower-level processes, etc.)? Have the sequence and interaction of these processes been made clear?

Have the criteria and methods been determined to ensure that processes proceed to their planned outputs (i.e. contributing to improved quality of life for patients) in an effective manner?

Who ensures that suitable resources are provided with the aim of improving the quality of life of patients?

Do the planned processes indicate where suitable documentation has to be made available in order that the processes can proceed in an effective manner?

Do the planned processes show what monitoring and measurements have to be made: where and when?

Have all the tests that patients undergo been clearly identified?

If outsourced products or services are used by clinicians in patient diagnosis and treatment, does the plan show how the outsourcing will be adequately controlled?

If outsourced products or services are used by other staff in connection with patient care, how is the outsourcing adequately controlled?

Does the patient process identify the final test(s) to be undertaken before a patient can be discharged from hospital?
Who has the responsibility for the decision to discharge a patient?

Do patient treatment plans give details of any follow-up activities on patients after discharge from hospital?

Do patient treatment plans identify what records are to be taken and maintained as patients make progress towards achieving an improved quality of life?

Do patient treatment plans indicate how the hospital might ensure that there is a continual improvement in the effectiveness of the quality management system?

Customer-related processes (ISO 9001, clause 7.2)

Determination of requirements related to the product (ISO 9001, clause 7.2.1)

The needs of patients are paramount. This is summarized by the requirement to achieve an improved quality of life for patients, whenever possible.

Do clinicians accede to the guidelines issued or available from bodies such as NICE and NSF?

Who is responsible for reviewing the diagnosis and the proposed treatment of patients, before a decision is made to treat a patient?
Is this done by a single consultant?
Are groups of consultants ever involved in such decision making?
Please show me examples.

Review of requirements related to the product (ISO 9001, clause 7.2.2)

Are the reviews and the follow-up discussions recorded?
Please show me examples.

Can I please see documented evidence of such reviews?

Do such reviews define the product or service adequately?
Have all requirements differing from those previously expressed been resolved?
Is the hospital able to meet the defined requirements?
Is there evidence that the reviews include consideration of required delivery dates, as defined by the contracts or orders?
Following each review process has the outcome been that product and/or service requirements are clearly defined?

Customer communication (ISO 9001, clause 7.2.3)

How does the hospital attempt to collect information on patient feedback?

How does it respond to patient complaints?
Does the hospital have guidelines on how to deal with patient complaints?
Is PALS in place and being adhered to?

Design and development (ISO 9001, clause 7.3)

This clause has been justifiably excluded (see Chapter 9).

Purchasing (ISO 9001, clause 7.4)

Purchasing process (ISO 9001, clause 7.4.1)

It is understood that NHS hospitals are subjected to central purchasing on many of the products that the hospital purchases, so the hospital has no direct control over the quality, price and delivery times of many purchased products.

What kinds of controls are exercised by the hospital over suppliers and subcontractors that can have a bearing on patient diagnosis or treatment, when it does have the freedom to make purchases other than through central purchasing?

What criteria are used for their selection?
Are evaluations carried out periodically?
If so, is this done at defined intervals?

Are records of the results of all evaluations kept and maintained as records?
Can I please see such records?

Can I please see any records of re-evaluations that have become necessary because of unsatisfactory product or poor service?

Has the introduction of purchasing controls resulted in a reduction in the number of suppliers and subcontractors, with consequential savings in administration?

Purchasing information (ISO 9001, clause 7.4.2)

Could I please see a few purchasing orders?

How are orders reviewed and approved to ensure the adequacy of specified purchase requirements before being despatched?
Please show me examples.

Verification of purchased product (ISO 9001, clause 7.4.3)

Is any purchased product examined before the time of its use?
If only certain products are examined before use, what criteria are used to determine what shall be examined on receipt?

In the case of a new supplier, does the hospital impose strict verification processes?
Are the strict verification processes agreed in advance and implemented on receipt of goods?
Please show me an example.

Production and service provision (ISO 9001, clause 7.5)

Control of production and service provision (ISO 9001, clause 7.5.1)

I need evidence that the hospital carries out patient diagnoses and treatment, as planned, under controlled conditions. Let us consider one or two patients.

Please can I see the case notes of several patients?

What patient processes were followed in the cases examined?

What equipment is being used?

What documentation is in place for this patient?

What monitoring and measuring devices are being used?

What requirements have to be satisfied before the patient can be discharged?

How does the hospital ensure that patients are handled carefully and safely at all times and in different circumstances?

Who is responsible for any patient follow-up activities?

Validation of processes for production and service provision (ISO 9001, clause 7.5.2)

This clause applies to those processes in which the resulting outcome cannot be directly validated.

Does the hospital have any processes, e.g. sterilization of instruments, for which only indirect validation of such processes is possible? (Such indirect validation must demonstrate the ability of the processes to achieve planned results.)

Have criteria been defined for review and approval of any such processes?

Has the equipment used been approved by a recognized authority?
Have personnel using the equipment been proved to be competent in the use of the equipment by a recognized authority?

Are specific methods and procedures being used that have been approved by recognized bodies?

Are appropriate records kept and maintained in this connection?

Whenever planned outcome is evidently not being achieved, does revalidation take place following appropriate changes to equipment, materials or staff?

Identification and traceability (ISO 9001, clause 7.5.3)

Identification

How are patients identified:

- in the A & E department?
- as in-patients?
- as day-patients?
- as out-patients?

What documentation is in place for this purpose?
Please show me examples.

Following any requirements to monitor and measure patients, during a patient process, who is responsible for recording such information and identifying the status of a patient? Please show me a few examples.

Traceability

In terms of patient diagnosis and treatment, does the hospital have to control and record the unique identification of any individual items, or batches of items, or hazardous patient processes?

If so, please show me how such traceability is achieved.
Please show me an example.

As far as other hospital services are concerned, does the hospital choose to identify and trace who did what and when so as to give full control over such services?
Please can I see examples?

Customer property (ISO 9001, clause 7.5.4)

Does the hospital have any documentation to help to ensure that all property belonging to a patient is properly controlled?
Please show me any such documentation.

What happens when patient property is lost or damaged?
Do you have strict guidelines in this connection?
Have you an example of such an incident that I can examine?

Preservation of product (ISO 9001, clause 7.5.5)

Identification

See clause 7.5.3.

Handling

Has the hospital issued guidelines on how to handle patients safely at all times?
Please may I see the guidelines?

Have similar guidelines been issued in connection with the handling of stock, equipment, etc?
Please may I see these guidelines too?

Packaging

What controls does the hospital have in place to ensure that any packing or packaging is adequate to prevent any damage that might occur and thereby result in a stock becoming unacceptable for use on patients?
Please show me examples.

What methods are used for identifying packaged stock?
Show me examples.

Once a product has been suitably identified, how is the identification preserved until it is delivered to the intended destination?

Storage

For stock awaiting use, do you have dedicated storage areas suitably organized so as to prevent damage or deterioration of stock whilst it is awaiting use?
Please show me examples.

How do you deal with incoming products that are likely to deteriorate with time?
Please show me examples.

Protection

How does the hospital provide protection for its patients from malicious damage and sexual assault whilst within the confines of the hospital?

How does the hospital provide protection for stock against damage, or theft, whilst within the confines of the hospital?

Preservation

Every effort is made whilst the patient is still in hospital to ensure that a patient's quality of life is not allowed to deteriorate in any way.

How does management ensure that this aspiration is always maintained?

On non-clinical matters, how does the hospital ensure that sensitive products, which might be damaged by any adverse method of packaging and storage, are preserved whilst under the hospital's control so that product remains undamaged from any such potential threats up to the time of its delivery for patient use?

In controlling stock, is consideration given to controlling environmental conditions, such as temperature, humidity, lighting and static electricity?

If damage by static electricity is a possibility, is special packaging and storage used to prevent electrostatic damage to stock?

Is all incoming stock carefully segregated and preserved until it is required for use?

Delivery

How does the hospital ensure that all patients are handled carefully to avoid injury whilst being moved within the hospital?

If patients are transferred to another hospital how does the hospital ensure that this is done safely?

Control of monitoring and measuring devices (ISO 9001, clause 7.6)

Clinicians decide what monitoring and measurements need to be made during patient diagnosis and treatment in order to achieve an improvement in the quality of life of their patients. In most cases the accuracy of any measurements with a given measuring device is unimportant and there is no need to have such devices calibrated.

However, if a clinician and/or another member of staff decides that a device needs to be calibrated (as opposed to being simply maintained) what arrangements are in place to ensure that calibration of devices is carried out properly?
If calibrations are required, who decides whether devices are to be calibrated externally or by hospital staff (i.e. internally)?

How are devices safeguarded from irresponsible adjustments that would invalidate the calibration?

How are devices protected from damage and deterioration during handling, maintenance and storage?

If a device is suspected to be out-of-calibration, or is found to be out-of-calibration at recalibration, who decides what are the possible consequences of the use of the device on patients diagnosed or treated earlier?

Is there a requirement to advise top management in all such cases?

If corrective actions need to be taken, who would be responsible for such action?
Is this documented?

Have patients ever been recalled to the hospital because of calibration problems?
If so, please show me the details.

If software is used in patient diagnosis and treatment, how is it validated prior to use?

External calibration

Are any devices calibrated externally?

Have UKAS accredited calibration laboratories been used?

If non-UKAS accredited laboratories have been used, has the equipment used to calibrate the hospital's equipment been calibrated by a UKAS calibration laboratory and thereby linked to an international or national standard?

Please can I examine all the hospital's external calibration certificates?

Does the hospital keep accurate records on all calibrations?
Please show me the records.
Is there a calibration register?

Does it state the calibration intervals for each device?

Does the hospital keep calibration logs for each piece of externally calibrated equipment?

Does the calibration register and the calibration logs show the normal locations of calibrated equipment so that, in the event that a calibration label is detached from a piece of calibrated equipment, its unique identification and calibration status can be traced through a process of elimination?

Which externally calibrated devices are to be used as reference standards?

Are devices used as reference standards set aside in a safe and secure environment and used only for internal calibrations?

Internal calibration

What are the acceptable limits for the calibration results for a particular instrument or device that is to be calibrated internally?

Is the known accuracy of the calibrated reference standard sufficiently greater (e.g. ten times greater) than the theoretical accuracy of the instrument or device being calibrated internally?

Is the uncertainty for the calibrated reference standard low enough to ensure that the uncertainty of calibration of the instrument or device being calibrated will be acceptable in the circumstances in which it will be used?

Who decides how often the instrument or device will need to be calibrated?

What documentation is used to ensure that all internal calibrations are carried out in a professional and scientifically acceptable manner?

Is the environment suitable for the calibrations being performed?

Who is responsible for internal calibrations?

Is documentation available for each device that is to be calibrated internally to ensure that all relevant matters are addressed and that the steps to be taken in the calibration process are clearly defined?

Unique identification of calibrated devices

Has all calibrated equipment (externally calibrated and internally calibrated) been uniquely identified?
How is this done?

If labelling is used, do labels give:

- a unique identification number, or code for the equipment?
- the date when calibration took place?
- the date when recalibration is due?
- the initials of the person responsible for calibration?

Are there unusual circumstances in which it was found impossible to place a label on calibrated equipment?
How is this identification problem overcome?

Measurement, analysis and improvement (ISO 9001, clause 8)

General (ISO 9001, clause 8.1)

There is a requirement on the hospital to plan and implement monitoring and measurement processes, analysis processes (with explanations of the methods used), and improvement processes in order to:

- ensure conformity of the quality management system to the requirements of ISO 9001;
- demonstrate a clinical requirement to improve the quality of life of patients and for other staff who provide all the other services in connection with patient care;
- continually improve the effectiveness of the quality management system.

Do you feel confident that the hospital has addressed these issues in general?

These specific requirements and associated requirements are addressed below.

Monitoring and measurement (ISO 9001, clause 8.2)

Customer satisfaction (ISO 9001, clause 8.2.1)

Does the hospital monitor patient satisfaction?

What methods are used to obtain information relating to patient perceptions as to whether the hospital has met patient requirements?

Have clinicians managed to achieve an improved quality of life for patients?
Have other staff provided a satisfactory service in terms of patient care?

How is the information obtained used to determine such patient perceptions?

Can I please see the latest findings?
Are they more satisfactory than earlier findings?

Internal audits (ISO 9001, clause 8.2.2)

What do you think is the purpose of internal audits?

The procedure internal audits must explain how internal audits are controlled.

The procedure, together with the quality manual, must answer the following questions.

Are the responsibilities and requirements for planning and conducting audits clearly stated?

Are the methods of reporting results clearly defined?

Does the procedure make clear how records will be kept and maintained?

May I please see your audit program?
Has consideration been given to the status and importance of the activities and areas to be audited, as well as the results of previous audits?

Does anyone audit his or her own work?

Please show me evidence that auditors have been trained.

Please may I see the records of a few internal audits?

How does management ensure that timely corrective action is taken on nonconformities and any observations found during the audit?
Please show me a few examples.

How is verification of any corrective actions and preventive actions achieved?

How are results recorded and reported to management?

Monitoring and measurement of processes (ISO 9001, clause 8.2.3)

How are all major and any lower-level processes monitored (and/or measured, as and when deemed necessary) so that:

- the clinical outputs eventually result in patients achieving an improved quality of life?
- other staff provide a continuing satisfactory service in connection with patient care?

Show me one example of monitoring and measurement undertaken during a patient process through the hospital.

If monitoring shows that a requirement is not being met, how is this dealt with?
Can you please show me examples of any such nonconformities found?

Monitoring and measurement of product (ISO 9001, clause 8.2.4)

How is the improved quality of life of patients monitored (and perhaps measured) to verify that planned changes have been achieved?

How are the services provided by non-clinical staff monitored (and perhaps measured) to determine whether the supporting services provided in connection with patient care conformed to planned arrangements?

Who has the authority to discharge patients (excluding those who discharge themselves)?

Control of nonconforming product (ISO 9001, clause 8.3)

(Important note: The failure of a patient to respond to treatment as expected is not to be regarded as a nonconformity, since treatment of patients is not an exact science. However, the failure to give the correct amount of a drug (wrongly prescribed, or carelessness on the part of a clinician), or the wrong injection of a drug into the spine, as opposed to being injected into the venous system, is to be regarded as a nonconformity, and recorded as such.)

The procedure control of nonconforming product, together with the quality manual, must answer the following questions.

When a patient fails to respond to treatment as expected, is this documented on the prescribed forms?
Who has the responsibility and authority to make decisions on future action?
Have nonconformities occurred in this respect (see note above)?

When supporting services in connection with patient care fail to operate as scheduled, or as planned, are such failures documented on the prescribed forms?
Who has the responsibility and authority to make decisions to prevent a reoccurrence of such failures?

How are any other unsatisfactory services (once identified) documented on the prescribed forms?

Are all nonconformities followed through as specified on the prescribed forms?

Who has the ultimate responsibility and authority to judge whether the action taken has been appropriate?

How do you ensure that a nonconforming service that has, allegedly, been corrected is subject to reverification after correction to demonstrate conformity?

What arrangements are in place to ensure that if a nonconformity in treatment, or in the provision of a service for a patient, is discovered after a patient has been discharged, or after attending hospital, then patients are advised accordingly and appropriate action is taken?

Analysis of data (ISO 9001, clause 8.4)

What data are collected and analysed:

- to demonstrate the effectiveness of the quality management system?
- to evaluate how continual improvements can be made in the effectiveness of the quality management system?

How are data analysed to provide information relating to:

- opportunities for corrective actions?
- opportunities for preventive actions?
- patient satisfaction?

Improvement (ISO 9001, clause 8.5)

Continual improvement (ISO 9001, clause 8.5.1)

How does the hospital continually improve the effectiveness of the quality management system?

One of the requirements of ISO 9001 is that an organisation should be striving at all times to improve continually (not continuously) the effectiveness of its quality management system. Can you give me examples of the ways in which the hospital has achieved any such improvements in the effectiveness of its quality management system?

Corrective action (ISO 9001, clause 8.5.2)

One of the mandatory procedures is on corrective action.
Please may I see it.

How are nonconformities and patient complaints identified?

How many have been recorded in each category over the last six months?

Is a log kept for each category?

Who is responsible for determining the cause of any nonconformities and patient complaints?
Please show me a number of different examples.

Who is responsible for determining the need for action(s) to ensure that nonconformities are corrected and patient complaints are addressed promptly?
Please show me a number of different examples.

Who is responsible for implementing appropriate corrective actions needed in both cases?
Please show me examples.

Who verifies the corrective actions taken?
Please show me examples.

Are corrective actions reviewed, for example, at management review meetings to ensure that they have been effective?
Please show me evidence of such reviews.

Preventive action (ISO 9001, clause 8.5.3)

One of mandatory procedures is on preventive action. Please may I see it?

Who is responsible for deciding when there is a need to take preventive action because of a nonconformity?

Who is responsible for deciding when there is a need to take preventive action because of a patient complaint?

Risk management

Does the hospital have a risk management committee?

How often does it meet?
Who is responsible for risk management?
Is there an overall risk management document?
Is the risk management document available to everyone?
Are risk management appraisals carried out and documented?

Contingency planning

What routine contingency planning for untoward events has taken place in relation to:

- cross-infection in the hospital?
- a health and safety policy?
  - Is there a health and safety document applicable to all employees?
  - Who is responsible for health and safety?
  - Is there an annual report on health and safety?
  - Are all employees trained in health and safety?
- a major incidents plan?
- a fire safety policy?
  - Are fire safety arrangements checked routinely?
- a waste disposal policy?
- disposal of clinical waste policy?
- security measures?
  - What arrangement exists for the safe-keeping of patients' belongings?
  - How is access to hospital buildings controlled?
  - How are staff identified?
  - What guidelines have been issued on physical and verbal abuse?
- control of drugs?

Risk assessments

Are risk assessments updated in the light of changed circumstances and untoward incidents?
Are untoward incidents, including clinical untoward incidents, and near misses fully documented for discussion at the risk management committee?
Are all such incidents reported to the National Patient Safety Agency?
Are risk analysis (RA) numbers determined for particular risks?
Who is responsible for deciding when there is a need to take preventive action because of a high RA number (or a high consequence rating associated with that number) for a particular activity in a hospital process?

Have other risk management techniques been used that have resulted in preventive actions being taken?
Can you please show me examples in each of the above cases in which preventive actions have been taken?

How does the hospital decide who will be responsible for implementing preventive actions?
Please show me examples.

Who verifies the preventive actions taken?
Please show me examples.

Are preventive actions reviewed, for example, at management review meetings to ensure that they have been effective?
Please show me evidence of such reviews.

Who is responsible for ensuring that appropriate hospital employees are made aware of the importance of preventing untoward events and the documentation that is in place for dealing with such events?

Does the personnel department keep records of all such training?

Additional Clinical audit guideline questions that can be incorporated into an ISO 9001 audit

Clinical audit schedule

I note that according to the clinical audit schedule for the hospital, this clinical audit is not on schedule. It is almost a month overdue.
Please can you explain this?
Did the chief executive give approval to the rescheduling?
If so, do you have a copy of the latest audit schedule?
If not, can you make me a copy please?

Patient process diagram

Does a patient process exist in the department in the form of a process diagram?
Does the patient process diagram refer to lower-level diagrams and/or notes that are applicable at different points of the process diagram?

Are all members of staff invited to suggest ways in which the patient process can be improved?
Can you please show me an example of this?
Is it available for everybody in the department to examine and follow?

In the preparation and revision of the department's patient process are comments made by patients, carers and other organizations devoted to the interests of patients taken into consideration?
Please give me an example of this.

Has the department patient process been approved by the head of the department and by top management?
How and when?

Is the patient process diagram reviewed on a systematic basis?

Is the department's patient process diagram issued to other departments that interface with the department?
Please show me examples of such referrals.

Internal documentation

Can I please see the list of documents that have been prepared for the department?

Do these include policies and procedures?

Some documents will be relevant across the entire hospital:

- risk management
- Patient Advisory and Liaison Service (PALS).

Please could I see a few examples of these reports, for example, the one entitled: 'How to minimize cross-infection in the hospital'?

Are all staff aware of the significance of the Patient Advisory and Liaison Service?
I would like to ask a few members of staff, now. May I?
(PALS does not fall under the remit of clinical audit, but under clinical governance. Nevertheless all staff must be aware of its significance.)

External documentation

Can I please see the list of external documents that are applicable to this department?

What national targets are in place for the work taking place in the department?
Please show me evidence that the department is striving to achieve these targets.

Are any NICE documents relevant?
If so, please show me examples.
Please show me evidence that the department is striving to adhere to such documents?

Are any NSF documents relevant?
If so, please show me examples.
Please show me evidence that the department is striving to adhere to such documents.

Are any NPSA documents relevant?
If so, please show me examples.
Please show me evidence that the department is striving to adhere to such documents.

Current clinical practice

Have any examples of the patient process not being followed?
When this happens is it recorded?
How is it recorded?
Is there a prescribed nonconformity form for such purposes?
Please may I see any such completed forms?

In the last six months, have you had any untoward events, adverse events or near miss events with patients?

Were they fully documented?
Please show me the documentation.
Was the chief executive advised immediately?

In the last six months, has anyone become aware of an unnecessary risk to patients that has not been realized hitherto?
Was a report made immediately to the chief executive?
If so, please show me.

I should now like to choose several patients at random. Please may I? Thank you.

Patient X

Please give me an overview of this patient, X.
Excellent. I have the picture. I note that you say the patient has already been discharged from hospital.

I should now like to sit down and examine all the relevant documents associated with this patient from the time of arrival to departure from hospital. Perhaps you could supplement what I read by answering a few questions from time to time?

(The purpose at this stage is to confirm, or otherwise, that the patient process and any relevant internal and external documentation was adhered to.)

I note that the outcome was apparently entirely satisfactory for the patient on leaving hospital.
Has the patient been back to a hospital out-patients' clinic?
If so, may I please see the notes made at the clinic?

Did anyone ask the patient for his views on the hospital experience and its outcome?
Were they recorded?
If so, please may I see the comments made?

Patient Z

Once again, please give me an overview. Thank you.

Since this patient is still in hospital, may I please see the patient? Thank you.
Is the patient in a fit enough state to answer a few simple questions?

Hello. I am so-and-so. Dr. … has kindly agreed to let me ask you a few questions. I am conducting what is called a clinical audit on this department and I would like to ask you a few simple questions. Have you any objections? If you have, I will go to another patient. Anything you say will be treated as being confidential and restricted to a very small number of people whose job it is to improve the stay of patients in the hospital.
Dr. … will leave us for a few moments. OK?
Thank you.

Can I ask whether as a patient you have always felt that your care, comfort and safety have evidently always been uppermost in the minds of those that have been in touch with you?

Have all staff been kind and considerate at all times?

Has your privacy always been respected?

Is the food good and delivered on time?

Do you feel that doctors and others try to explain to you what they are doing and what they intend to do?

Is there anything at all that you feel I should know about that in your opinion should not happen to patients?

Thank you for your help.

The audit on this patient is then concluded in the same way as for patient X, except that the outcome is not yet known since the patient is still in hospital.

Other patients

Depending on the time still available other patient processes, outcomes and experiences can be examined.

Improvements in clinical practice

What changes have been made in clinical practice since the last clinical audit?

In the absence of a previous clinical audit what changes have been made to clinical practice during the last six months?
Please can I see the documentation in connection with those changes?

Benefits to patients of changes in clinical practice

Are you sure that patients have benefited from the changes in clinical practice?
Please give me a few examples.

Data collection and analysis

What data are collected on patient diagnosis, treatment and outcomes?
Can I please see examples?

What data are collected about the patient experience on timings: time between referral by a GP and first hospital appointment; the time, for example, to determine that routine surgery is necessary; the time waiting for surgery; cancellation of surgery appointments; time of actual surgery; time between first referral and time of actual surgery?
Please show me examples of any such data.
Do the data satisfy government targets?

How is such data on many patients collated and analysed?
Can I please see examples?

Are all data, collations of data and analyses of data submitted routinely to top management for discussion?
Have the discussions within departments and with top management resulted in improvements?
Can you please give me an example of such improvements as a result of the collection, collation and analysis of such data?

How does such data and analyses on patient diagnosis, treatment and outcomes, and on timings, compare with similar data and analyses from other hospitals?
Are the data and analyses submitted to NICE and other relevant bodies?
Please can I see such comparisons?
Have any discrepancies been satisfactorily explained?
Please can I see such evidence?

Appendix 1: Quality management system mandatory procedures

This appendix includes the mandatory procedures for ISO 9001. It is recommended that any other procedures, mandatory or otherwise, follow the same format. The mandatory procedures are as follows.

PC 101	Control of Documents
PC 102	Control of Records
PC 103	Internal Audit
PC 104	Control of Nonconforming Product
PC 105	Corrective Action
PC 106	Preventive Action

Quality Management System Procedure

Control of Documents

Controlled Copy

Copy no: ....

Registered holder: ....

Position: ....

Prepared by: .... Approved by: ....

Management representative

Date: .... Supersedes: ....

PC 101 Issue 1

1. Purpose

The purpose of this procedure is to show how the documents are controlled within the quality management system.

The rigid controls that are imposed on such documents are there for a specific purpose, namely, to ensure that only approved latest issues of documents are in use in appropriate locations throughout the hospital.

2. Scope

This procedure applies to all the documents within the quality management system. The framework documentation includes:

- the quality manual;
- process diagrams;
- procedures;
- policies;
- forms;
- templates;
- external documents;
- external forms.

Working documents (see Chapter 4) will include some of the following:

- patient case notes;
- X-ray films, scans, etc;
- protocols;
- clinical forms and templates;
- clinical external documents;
- clinical forms.

Other documents can be created as deemed necessary by heads of departments.

3. Responsibilities

The process of changing and controlling framework documents within the quality management system is managed by the management representative. The management representative must also be satisfied that working documents are controlled in a systematic manner.

4. Associated documents

Forms:

FM 101	Control of Framework Documentation
FM 102	Acceptance of Documentation
FM 103	Register of Framework Documentation
FM 104	Framework documentation – Change Request
FM 105	Changes to Framework Documentation

5. Details of procedure

5.1 Control of documents

The management representative is responsible for giving final approval to all documents that are part of the hospital's quality management system.

It is inevitable that some documents will have to be changed from time to time. These must be reapproved by the management representative prior to being reissued to interested parties.

Changes to external documents and external forms cannot be made by the hospital, but the management representative has the responsibility of ensuring that they are properly controlled.

5.2 Reference letters and numbers, issue numbers and revision numbers

5.2.1 Reference letters and numbers

The reference letters that precede reference numbers, issue numbers and revision numbers have been allocated as follows:

QM	quality management system policy manual;
PD	process diagram;
PC	procedure;
PT	protocol;
WI	work instruction;
PL	policies
FM	form;
EFM	external form;
ED	external document.

The appendices to the quality manual provide useful information as an important part of the quality manual, but they can also be used as stand-alone documents.

External forms and external documents need to be considered as part of the quality management system documentation and properly controlled, as they might have some bearing on the quality of the services provided by the hospital.

Each document is given a unique reference number, e.g. 101, which follows the reference letters. In some cases blocks of numbers, e.g. 101 to 150, are allocated to certain departments or certain activities.

5.2.2 Issue and revision numbers

The issue number of a document is indicated by an appendage 1, 2, 3, etc. An original page does not have a revision status, but if a single page is altered in any way it is given a revision appendage, e.g. Rev. 1, which indicates the first revision status of a page. Further revisions of the same page become Rev. 2, Rev. 3, etc.

When a number of pages have undergone revision, the document can be reissued without revision numbers, but with the grading of issue 2, issue 3, etc. The management representative decides when this will be done.

Forms do not have revision numbers, only issue numbers.

External forms and external documents are listed in a logical manner by the management representative.

5.3 Distribution of documents

Each copy of the quality manual or a procedure is given a unique copy number. When controlled documents are despatched to a member of staff, they are accompanied by FM 101. An Acceptance of Documentation form, FM 102, will also be sent. This must be signed by the recipient and returned to the management representative.

When, for instance, a procedure is reissued following a number of changes, the superseded documents must be returned to the management representative. Single pages that have been superseded must be destroyed by the recipient of the new pages. Such measures should prevent the continuing use of superseded documents. If the management representative decides to keep superseded documents for knowledge preservation purposes or for any other reasons, they are clearly identified by a stamp as being 'superseded'.

It is the responsibility of the head of a unit or department to ensure that relevant versions of applicable documents are always available at points of use. Such documents must remain legible and be readily identifiable.

The appendices to the quality manual will change from time to time; these will be issued to recipients in a controlled manner.

Documents of external origin are listed by the management representative. They are distributed, and updated when necessary, in the same manner as any other documents. This ensures that only the latest version of any external document, or external form, is being used.

The management representative uses form FM 103 to keep a record of where documents are.

5.4 Changes to documents

All staff are encouraged to make suggestions on how to improve the documents on which the hospital's quality management system is based. Any such changes should first be discussed with immediate colleagues who might be affected by the proposed changes.

Requests for any changes should be made on a Change Request form, FM 104. This is submitted to the management representative who, after due consultation with interested parties and perhaps discussion in a management review meeting, may issue an amendment to the documentation.

Changes in a document are identified by a vertical line placed in the left hand margin, alongside the changed line(s) or paragraph(s). When a page is changed in this way, the revision number is increased as explained above. When a further change is made on the same page, only the latest change is indicated by a vertical line.

When a number of changes have been made to a document, the management representative may decide to reprint and redistribute the document with a new issue number (with no revision number).

Form FM 105 is also issued to staff along with any changes to the documents. Such forms summarize the changes made to a particular document, including the latest changes. They are intended to be retained as an appendix to the document in question, so that anyone can see what changes have been made. As appendices, they are placed at the back of the relevant part of the documentation.

5.5 Quality management system forms

A complete set of controlled forms will be held in several designated places within the hospital. They can be copied for use as and when necessary.

Changes to forms are addressed in the same way as changes to any other documents.

5.6 Uncontrolled documents

Each controlled document is stamped 'controlled copy' in red ink. Copying of the framework documentation is not normally allowed, with the exception of external documents and external forms, since such uncontrolled copies would defeat the objective of maintaining controls on the quality management system documentation. Uncontrolled documents can easily be identified, as the red 'controlled copy' stamp will either be absent or not be red. Nevertheless, occasionally, there may be a need for extra copies of a document to be available, e.g. for discussion purposes at a meeting. If such a need arises, copies may be made with the approval of the management representative, but each copy should be clearly stamped 'Uncontrolled'. The uncontrolled copies should be withdrawn from circulation as soon as practicable.

In the case of uncontrolled copies that are issued in formulating a quality plan, the uncontrolled copies may become an integrated part of the quality plan and as such will need to remain in situ perhaps for some considerable time, if the quality plan becomes dormant. However, when such a quality plan is reactivated, the project manager will obtain from the management representative a controlled copy of the relevant document and the uncontrolled copy will be returned.

5.7 Documents (and records) on computer

Many documents and records (see PC 102) are stored on computer. The same rules apply to electronic storage as apply to storage of hard copy documents and records, but additional safeguards are required: back-up storage, prevention of unauthorized access to data, as well as prevention of data corruption.

The management representative has to be satisfied that adequate controls are in place for these purposes.

5.8 Bureaucratic documentation

The quality management system documentation must not be bureaucratic. If any member of staff believes that a document serves little or no useful purpose, such thoughts should be aired with colleagues with a view to getting the bureaucratic document amended or removed from the quality management system via the management representative.

Control of Framework Documentation

To: ....

Listed below, and attached hereto, are controlled documents for your retention. Please ensure that the documents are accessible to your colleagues so that there can be no misunderstanding as to how the hospital functions.

....

....

....

....

....

....

....

....

....

....

....

....

....

....

I shall be glad to receive any suggestions for improving the documentation.

Please sign and return the attached form (FM 102). If you are receiving a document which supersedes an existing one, please ensure that you return the superseded document at the same time.

Date: ....

Management representative: ....

FM 101 Issue 1.

Acceptance of Documentation

To: the management representative

I accept the safe receipt of the following controlled documents:

....

....

....

....

....

....

I am returning the following superseded documents:

....

....

....

....

....

....

....

....

I shall be glad to receive any suggestions for improving the documentation.

If you are receiving a document which supersedes an existing one, please ensure that you return the supersede document at the same time.

Date: ....

Recipient: ....

FM 102 Issue 1.

Register of Framework Documentation

Reference no.	Name	Date issued	Date acknow-ledgement returned	Superseded documents that have been returned	Signature of management representative

FM 103 Issue 1. Page of

Framework Documentation – Change Request

Reference:
Proposed change:
Requested by: .... Date: .... Position: .... Department: ....
Comments sought from: Comments by reviewer(s): Signature(s) of reviewer(s): .... Date: ....
Approved/rejected by management representative: .... Date: ....

FM 104 Issue 1.

Changes to Framework Documentation

Reference no.	Amendment/additions	Date issued	Signature of management representative

FM 105 Issue 1.

Page of

Quality Management System Procedure

Control of Records

Controlled Copy

Copy no: ....

Registered holder: ....

Position: ....

Prepared by: .... Approved by: ....

Management representative

Date: .... Supersedes: ....

PC 102 Issue 1

1. Purpose

The purpose of this procedure is to ensure that records are established and maintained to prove that the quality management system is in place and working effectively, in accordance with hospital's quality policy and in pursuance of hospital's quality objectives.

2. Scope

This procedure applies to all the documents specified below and to others subsequently named by the relevant managers and the quality manager in the light of experience.

3. Responsibilities

The quality manager is responsible for ensuring that records are collected, suitably filed and stored. Responsibility for records in the first instance lies with clinicians, other professional staff, managers and their staff, who create and use the records. All staff are expected to contribute, directly or indirectly, towards the establishment and maintenance of records during their everyday activities.

4. Associated documents

These are too diverse to list individually, since records arise from many quality management system documents and from day-to-day operations.

5.0 Details of procedure

5.1 Quality records

Records arise from the many activities that occur in the hospital. They provide objective evidence of what has happened.

ISO 9001:2000 requires, as a minimum, that certain records specified in the standard are established, kept and maintained. These are records on the following:

(a) management review meetings (see clause 5.6.1);

(b) education, training, skills and experience [see clause 6.2.2 (e)];

(c) to provide evidence that realization processes and their results meet planned arrangements [see clause 7.1 (d)], i.e. the hospital will establish and maintain day-to-day patient records that are key to proving what happened, where and when. One copy is retained in the patient's case notes;

(d) results of reviews of patient's needs and the actions arising from these reviews (see clause 7.2.2);

(e) results from the evaluation of suppliers (except for central purchases) and the necessary actions arising from the evaluations (see clause 7.4.1);

(f) validation of processes where the resulting output cannot be verified by subsequent monitoring or measurement, e.g. as is the case with sterilization equipment [see clause 7.5.2 (d)];

(g) unique identification of patients and products (e.g. drugs) (see clause 7.5.3);

(h) results of any calibrations on equipment, if applicable (see clause 7.6);

(i) validity of any previous measurements when measuring equipment is found to be, or suspected of being, out of calibration (see clause 7.6);

(j) results of internal audits and actions arising thereafter (see clause 8.2.2);

(k) person(s) responsible for authorizing the release of patients (see clause 8.2.4);

(l) nonconformities (see clause 8.3);

(m) corrective actions and their signing-off (see clause 8.5.2);

(n) patient complaints and their outcomes (see clause 8.5.2);

(o) preventive actions and their effectiveness (see clause 8.5.3).

In addition a hospital should establish and maintain the records on:

(p) changes to the quality management system's documentation (see PC 101);

(q) documentation relating to assessments and surveillances by a certification body;

(r) monitoring of patient satisfaction;

(s) contracts;

(t) maintenance carried out within the hospital that might have a bearing on the quality of patient care and the services provided for patients;

(u) quality plans and other documents that are considered relevant to the care of patients;

(v) review of quality objectives;

(w) review of quality policy (as and when deemed necessary);

(x) any other records that management and/or clinicians deem should be kept for statutory reasons and/or for continuing quality care of patients.

5.2 Collection, care and collation of records

Everyone associated with the creation of records must ensure that the records are:

- readily identified;
- legible and remain legible;
- stored appropriately;
- protected from damage;
- easy to retrieve.

The quality manager is responsible for the collection and collation of records arising directly from the quality management system documents. They also have to be satisfied that clinicians and other professional staff are collecting and collating their records in a satisfactory manner.

Storage will initially take place in designated areas following discussion with appropriate staff. Longer term storage will also be decided in consultation with the quality manager.

Once a year the quality manager, clinicians and other designated people have to confirm in writing to the management review committee that all the defined records are in place, properly filed and preserved.

Many records are stored on computer. The rules that apply to hard copy records also apply to those stored electronically, but additional safeguards are required, e.g. back-up storage, prevention of unauthorized access to data, and prevention of data corruption (see PC 101).

5.3 Filing of quality records

All records are filed appropriately, but securely.

5.4 Access to records

Access to records will be restricted to senior staff and those who need to have access because of their day-to-day responsibilities. Any patient has the right to examine his or her own records.

5.5 Maintenance of records

The quality manager is responsible for maintaining the records directly associated with the quality management system. Likewise, clinicians and other staff who have responsibilities for initiating records based on their day-to-day activities are also responsible for their upkeep and safe storage.

5.6 Archiving of records

All hospital records will be archived from time to time by the quality manager, or a nominated person, in a manner that will allow easy traceability and retrieval when required.

Patient records are kept and maintained in a sound condition for a minimum period of seven years, from the date of the patient's last attendance at the hospital.

5.7 Disposal of quality records

The disposal of hospital records will be necessary from time to time. Only the chief executive in consultation with the quality manager can give approval for the disposal of records after the defined retention times have been exceeded.

More and more hospitals are tending to place patient records on microfiche so that the need for disposal of patient records is becoming increasingly irrelevant.

Quality Management System Procedure

Internal Audit

Controlled Copy

Copy no: ....

Registered holder: ....

Position: ....

Prepared by: .... Approved by: ....

Management representative

Date: .... Supersedes: ....

PC 103 Issue 1

1. Purpose

The purpose of this procedure is to explain how internal audits are conducted on all aspects of the hospital's quality management system with a view to establishing that:

- the quality management system conforms to the requirements of ISO 9001:2000;
- the quality management system conforms to the planned arrangements that aim to give patients a better quality of life;
- the quality management system is being effectively implemented and maintained.

The internal audits are intended to highlight any problems or difficulties and afford an opportunity to make approved changes.

2. Scope

This procedure applies to all the internal auditing activities that are undertaken by or on behalf of the hospital.

3. Responsibilities

It is the responsibility of the quality manager, or a person nominated by the chief executive and acting on their behalf, to ensure that internal auditing is carried out satisfactorily.

4. Associated documents

Quality management system manual

Forms:

Internal Audit Schedule, FM 121

Register of Internal Audits, FM 122

Internal Audit Questionnaire, FM 123

Nonconformity or Observation Form, FM 124

Summary – Internal Audit Report, FM 125

5.0 Details of procedure

5.1 General

Internal auditing is one of the most important aspects of the hospital's quality management system. It should be viewed in a positive manner, like patient complaints, because internal quality auditing affords an opportunity to the person being audited, and for the auditor carrying out the audit, to consider ways of improving how the hospital functions for the benefit of its patients.

5.2 Auditors

All auditing will be conducted by auditors who have received training in auditing. No auditor is allowed to audit their own work, but auditors can audit work for which they are responsible. Thus, a manager of a division can audit the work of the people working for them, but the manager cannot audit the actual work that they do. This could be done by, say, another manager in the hospital.

5.3 Planning of internal audits

The quality manager ensures that there is a comprehensive schedule for internal auditing that embraces all aspects of work carried out in the hospital. Such audits are carried out at least once a year. Areas of work that are important to the hospital's activities may undergo internal auditing at more frequent intervals. In addition, when an audit identifies problems, re-auditing will be arranged in the near future on an agreed date. The overall schedule for internal audits throughout the hospital is available for all members of staff to examine.

During the implementation of the quality management system, internal quality audits can be carried out as soon as an activity is considered to be ready for an audit. Proper records of findings are made of all audits, including these preliminary ones.

The internal audit schedule is shown on form FM 121. This form shows the dates on which internal audits will be conducted in different areas of the hospital. The form identifies processes and/or activities to be audited and the corresponding relevant areas of the standard.

Audits can be delayed or postponed in exceptional circumstances, but only with the approval of the chief executive and the quality manager. Additional audits will be arranged by the quality manager in consultation with heads of departments when a previous audit has proved to be unsatisfactory.

5.4 Internal audit register

Prior to any audit, the quality manager will allocate a number to an audit and also record the actual date of the audit on the Register of Internal Audits, FM 122. All subsequent documents associated with the particular audit will include the audit number and date.

The quality manager is responsible for maintaining the register at all times so that the status of internal audits can be readily determined at any given time.

5.5 Audit questions

Prior to any audit, an auditor will prepare a number of possible questions (Internal Audit Questionnaire, FM 123) in connection with the area being audited. These will form the basis of the audit but other questions may be asked in the light of what is subsequently revealed to an auditor.

It has been made clear to all staff that any one of them may be asked questions during an audit in order for the auditor to determine whether the quality management system documentation (for a process, procedure or work instruction) is being implemented satisfactorily and whether it is effective.

5.6 Findings of internal audits

Whenever an auditor discovers that there is a discrepancy (e.g. against a requirement of the standard or a process, procedure or work instruction) between what is laid down and what is actually taking place in a ward or area of work, objective evidence to this effect will be recorded on an internal audit Nonconformity or Observation Form, FM 124. The auditee will be asked to sign the form, thus indicating their agreement with the findings.

If the auditor, or the auditee, makes observations with a view to continual improvement of the effectiveness of the quality management system, such observations will be recorded on the same form, FM 124, and the word 'Nonconformity' at the top shall be crossed out.

At the end of the audit this form is sent to the quality manager after issues related to corrective and preventive action have been addressed.

5.7 Corrective action

The audit Nonconformity or Observation Form, FM 124, will need other entries. Someone, for instance, will have to state on the form what corrective action is to be taken. On occasions this may have to be completed after an audit for very good reasons. The person responsible for such action has to be named and their signature obtained. The date by which the changes are to be implemented also has to be given (see PC 105).

5.8 Preventive action

If preventive action is to be taken, it must be entered on the form. The person responsible for such action has to be named and their signature obtained. The date by which the changes are to be implemented also has to be given (see PC 106).

5.9 Verification of corrective and preventive action

It is the responsibility of the quality manager to add his signature to the form once verification of the corrective action, and possibly preventive action, has been confirmed.

5.10 Summary of internal audit

The auditor will complete a Summary – Internal Audit Report (FM 125) after each audit, in which the main findings (nonconformities and observations) are recorded along with an overall summary of the audit.

At the end of the audit, all of the Internal Audit Report forms (FM 125) are sent to the quality manager.

5.11 Completion of register of internal audits

After completion of an internal audit, the quality manager will enter the relevant information in the Register of Internal Audits (FM 122). If no nonconformities/observations have been found the form can be signed off immediately; otherwise, the audit will be 'signed off' only when the quality manager is satisfied that the actions have been completed satisfactorily.

5.12 Management reviews

The internal audit reports are considered at each management review meeting. They are used as the basis for any discussions on the successful implementation of the hospital's quality management system.

The management review committee has the authority to introduce changes via the quality manager with a view to continually improve the effectiveness of the quality management system.

5.13 Quality records

All the documents associated with internal audits will form part of the hospital's quality records. These will be retained for a minimum period specified by the chief executive.

Eventually, nonconformity reports will all be filed consecutively, but as an interim measure all outstanding nonconformity reports will be filed together in one group. As each outstanding corrective action (and possibly preventive action) is signed off by the quality manager, the report will be transferred to its appropriate sequential position in the 'closed off' section of the file.

Internal Audit Schedule, 2006

	Planned month Actual month	Jan	Feb	Mar	Apr	May	June	July	Aug	Sept	Oct	Nov	Dec
	Planned date Actual date												
ISO 9001 clause no.	Process/activity Reference process diagrams and/or Name of the relevant clause												

Nonconformities/observations indicated by N and/or O in appropriate box. When an audit has been cleared satisfactorily the box is ticked.

Date: ____________________ Signature of management representative: ....

FM 121 Issue 1. Page of

Register of internal audits

Audit no.	Date of audit	Activity reference document(s)	Completion date for corrective action(s)	Completion date for preventative action(s)	Signature of management representative following verification

FM 122 Issue 1.

Page of

Internal Audit Questionnaire

Audit no: ____________________ Process/activity/reference documents: ____________________

Manual, process, procedure, form	ISO 9001 reference	Question	Comments

FM 123 Issue 1.

Page of

Nonconformity or Observation Form

Audit no: .... Nonconformity or Observation no: ....

Process/activity audited	Reference documents	Date

Nonconformity or observation (cross out as appropriate):

Auditor: .... Signature: ....

Departmental representative: .... Signature: ....

<u>Nonconformity</u> – corrective action(s) proposed or <u>Observation</u> – resulting in continual improvements:

Person responsible for corrective action(s) or improvements: .... Signature: ....

Date by which corrective action(s) or improvements will be implemented: ....

Preventive action(s) proposed (write N/A if no preventive action is proposed):

Person responsible for preventive action(s): .... Signature: ....

Date by which preventive action(s) will be implemented:

Verification of corrective action(s) and preventive action(s)/adoption or rejection of observation

Signature of management representative: .... Date: ....

FM 124 Issue 1.

Page of

Summary – Internal Audit Report

Audit no: ....

Process/activity audited	Reference documents	Date

Nonconformities:

Observations:

Overall summary:
Auditor (print name): .... Signature: ....

FM 125 Issue 1.

Page of

Quality Management System Procedure

Control of Nonconforming Product

Controlled Copy

Copy no: ....

Registered holder: ....

Position: ....

Prepared by: .... Approved by: ....

Management representative

Date: .... Supersedes: ....

PC 104 Issue 1

1. Purpose

The purpose of this procedure is to ensure that all nonconformities are properly documented.

Although there is no mention of a procedure to deal with nonconformities arising from internal audits (see clause 8.2.2), the same basic procedure is followed when any nonconformities arise from them. Similarly, when nonconformities are discovered in any process (see clause 8.2.3), they too are addressed by the methods described in this procedure.

Whenever a hospital fails to abide by protocols or procedures, this procedure on nonconformities should be followed.

2. Scope

This procedure applies to all nonconformities with one exception.

The failure of a patient to respond to treatment as expected is not to be regarded as a nonconformity since treatment of patients is not an exact science. However, the failure of a clinician to administer a treatment (i.e. the correct amount of a drug) is to be regarded as a nonconformity and recorded as such.

3. Responsibilities

It is the responsibility of the quality manager to ensure that all nonconformities are dealt with in the manner prescribed in this procedure.

4. Associated documents

Forms:

Register of Internal Audits, FM 122

Nonconformity or Observation Form, FM 124

Register of Nonconformities, FM 131

Nonconformity Form, FM 132

5 Details of procedure

5.1 Nonconformities

All nonconformities in patient care are properly recorded and the nature of the nonconformity clearly explained. The name of the person who has caused any nonconformity, whatever their position, is clearly recorded on form FM 132. In some cases the cause of nonconformity is not the result of an individual's action or inaction. Any nonconformity in relation to patient care must be clearly identified and the nature of the nonconformity is recorded on a prescribed form. In addition, the nonconformity in patient care, once identified, results in a more carefully controlled process once the shortcoming has been identified.

Nonconformity in patient care must always result in action that deals with the results of the nonconformity. A record must be kept of the corrective action taken (FM 132). The quality manager must be kept fully informed. Only when the quality manager, or equivalent person, is satisfied that the nonconformity has been dealt with satisfactorily will the form be signed-off. It is retained as a record (see PC 102).

The effects of the corrective action taken for the benefit of a patient must be subject to a re-examination of a patient to ensure that the action taken has been effective.

If the hospital becomes aware of a nonconformity in patient care after a patient has left hospital, it must take appropriate action regarding the consequences, or potential consequences, of the nonconformity.

Exactly the same procedure is followed in the case of outsourced processes immediately after a nonconformity has been found.

5.2 Review of causes of nonconformities

Nonconformities will arise for many reasons in any organization: human failure; incompetence; disregard for procedures or other documentation, or an impractical protocol, procedure or process, etc., which has not been properly tried and tested before its introduction.

All factual information on nonconformities must be reviewed immediately after their discovery to ascertain the cause of nonconformities.

5.3 Prevention of repetition of a nonconformity

It is important to ensure that there is not a repetition of a nonconformity. The fourth part of the form FM 132 should be completed, if possible, perhaps after discussion with the other interested parties, to prevent a reoccurrence of the nonconformity. In those cases in which a single human failing has caused the nonconformity 'N/A' (not applicable) can be written in this section.

5.4 Verification of any corrective actions and any further actions

Form FM 132 is handed to the quality manager as soon as possible. On receipt they will allocate the next serial number to the form.

The quality manager will sign the last section of the form once they are satisfied that any corrective and preventive action has been carried out satisfactorily.

5.5 Register of nonconformities

The quality manager is responsible for maintaining a Register of Nonconformities, FM 131.

5.6 Filing of nonconformities

A file will be maintained for nonconformities. The file will be divided into two parts: the first part will contain active nonconformities, and the second will contain those that are closed.

5.7 Management review meetings

Top management reviews all such factual information on nonconformities. The quality manager will present all the different kinds of nonconformities that have been recorded since the last meeting. If there are nonconformities that still have to be signed off or closed from the last meeting, then it will be decided what action needs to be taken to do this.

Top management should be in a position to manage the hospital if:

(a) nonconformities are identified;

(b) the reasons for the nonconformities are identified,

(c) appropriate corrective, and perhaps preventive, action is taken; and

(d) the information in (a), (b) and (c) is fully documented.

5.8 Quality records

All the documentation associated with nonconformities will form part of the hospital's quality records.

Records on nonconformities will be maintained for a minimum period of time as specified by the chief executive.

Register of Nonconformities

No.	Product and/or service	Date discovered	Signature of management representative following corrective/preventive action

FM 131 Issue 1.

Page of

Nonconformity Form

No: ....

Patient: ....

Telephone no: ....

Reference no: .... Internal ref. no: ....

Nature of nonconformity:

Signature: .... Date discovered: ....

Corrective action(s) taken:

Person responsible
for corrective action(s): ....

Date: .... Signature: ....

Preventive action(s) proposed:

Person responsible
for preventive action(s): .... Signature: ....

Date by which preventive action(s) will be implemented: ....

Verification of corrective action(s) and preventive action(s)

Signature of management
representative: .... Date: ....

FM 132 Issue 1.

Quality Management System Procedure

Corrective Action
(arising from nonconformities and patient complaints)

Controlled Copy

Copy no: ....

Registered holder: ....

Position: ....

Prepared by: .... Approved by: ....

Management representative

Date: .... Supersedes: ....

PC 105 Issue 1

1. Purpose

The purpose of this procedure is to ensure that corrective action is taken to eliminate the cause of a nonconformity, or a patient complaint, in order to correct what is going wrong or what has gone wrong.

Corrective action must always be appropriate to the impact of the problem encountered and the likelihood of it reoccurring. For example, if a nonconformity or complaint is considered to be a one–off event with a very low probability of it happening again then a large amount of money correcting it needn't be spent.

On the other hand, if it is thought that the same or similar nonconformity or complaint might happen again sometime in the future, additional action (preventive action) might be taken to ensure that it does not reoccur. Sometimes, such preventive action might become part of the corrective action, if the action taken is greater than the essential corrective action necessary to put right what was going wrong or had gone wrong. In general it is better to think of corrective and preventive action as being distinct and separate. Corrective actions demand immediate attention: a nonconformity might have serious consequences, especially in a hospital, and patient complaints must be addressed without delay. Preventive actions should be implemented as soon as possible (see PC 106).

2. Scope

This procedure applies to all nonconformities and patient complaints.

3. Responsibilities

It is the responsibility of the quality manager to ensure that all corrective actions are dealt with in an expeditious manner and that appropriate documentation is raised.

4. Associated documents

Forms:

- Register of Internal Audits, FM 122
- Register of Nonconformities, FM 131
- Register of Patient Complaints, FM 141
- Nonconformity or Observation Form, FM 124
- Nonconformity Form, FM 132
- Patient Complaint Form, FM 142

Patient Advisory and Liaison Service (PALS) (see Appendix 3)

5. Details of procedure

5.1 Corrective action in response to nonconformities

Corrective action is essentially a backwards looking phenomenon, starting at the latest from the time that a decision is made that corrective action is necessary in order to put right what is going wrong or what has gone wrong. The implementation of the corrective action may not always be possible immediately, but it will take place as soon as possible or as appropriate in the immediate future.

Once a nonconformity has been identified, it is recorded on prescribed forms FM 124 and FM 132, as explained in procedures PC 103, PC 104 and this procedure.

The person who accepts responsibility for the corrective action must sign the form. All the forms referred to above include space for preventive action (see PC 106).

Finally, the prescribed form should be signed off only by a responsible person within the organization, usually the quality manager, when they are satisfied that the nonconformity has been satisfactorily dealt with from every point of view and the actions taken have been completed in every respect.

The corrective action taken should also be reviewed to decide whether it has been effective in dealing with the nonconformity.

All nonconformities are entered on the nonconformities register FM 131 and all nonconformity forms (FM 124 and 132) are systematically filed (see PC 104).

5.2 Patient complaints

There should be no doubt within a hospital about what is meant by a patient complaint. If anyone in the hospital feels that it is necessary to apologize to a patient, because they appear to be aggrieved by what has happened (or by what has not happened), then a complaint has been received. It may appear to be an unjustifiable complaint, but the patient evidently thinks otherwise, so it is advisable to be cautious and to promise to investigate the complaint without delay.

There are two important points to bear in mind when dealing with patient complaints. Firstly, the complaint must be addressed quickly and if it appears to be a serious complaint, it should be referred without delay to a senior member of staff for urgent action. Secondly, since 1 April 2002, all NHS hospitals have introduced the Patient Advisory and Liaison Service (PALS) (see Appendix 3) and its requirements must always be addressed.

5.3 Corrective action in response to patient complaints

A Patient Complaint Form, FM 142, similar to the Nonconformity Form FM 132, is used to deal with every complaint. Every complaint must be recorded on the prescribed form, whether it is a verbal complaint or a complaint made by telephone, fax, E-mail or letter. The form identifies the patient who has complained, the date and time of its receipt, the recipient of the complaint, and the nature of the complaint. The form includes space to state the corrective action taken. The person who accepts responsibility for the corrective action must sign that part of the form.

The form includes space for preventive action (see PC 106). The quality manager will sign the last section of the form once the complaint process has been completed.

As was the case for nonconformities, the quality manager is responsible for maintaining the Register of Patient Complaints (FM 141). All Patient Complaint Forms (FM 141 and FM 142) are systematically filed (see PC 104).

5.4 Management review meetings

At each management review meeting, the quality manager will present details of all nonconformities and patient complaints and the hospital's responses.

Such meetings will consider what action to take about the nonconformities that were reported at the last meeting that still have to be signed off.

All patient complaints should have been addressed promptly. Management should look upon patient complaints in a positive manner. They are not be used to ostracize people, although when incompetence has become evident, appropriate action needs to be taken by top management.

Most patients usually accept mistakes with good grace, provided corrective action is taken promptly. From the hospital's point of view, patient goodwill is thereby usually retained, adverse publicity is avoided and litigation is less likely.

5.5 Quality records

All the documentation associated with corrective actions taken in connection with nonconformities and patient complaints form part of the hospital's quality records.

Register of Patient Complaints

No.	Patient complaint	Date discovered	Date and signature of management representative following verification

FM 141 Issue 1. Page of

Patient Complaint Form

No: ....

Patient complaint:

Contact person: .... Telephone no: ....

Person's reference no: .... Internal no: ....

Nature of complaint:

Signature: .... Date : ....

Corrective action(s) taken: Justified/unjustified

Person responsible
for corrective action(s): ....

Date: .... Signature : ....

Preventive action(s) proposed (if any):

Person responsible
for preventive action(s): .... Signature: ....

Date by which preventive action(s) will be implemented: ....

Verification of corrective action(s) and preventive action(s)

Signature of management
representative: .... Date: ....

FM 142 Issue 1.

Quality Management System Procedure

Preventive Action
(arising from nonconformities,
patient complaints and risk management)

Controlled Copy

Copy no: ....

Registered holder: ....

Position: ....

Prepared by: .... Approved by: ....

Management representative

Date: .... Supersedes: ....

PC 106 Issue 1

1. Purpose

The purpose of this procedure is to ensure that preventive action is taken:

(i) to reduce the likelihood of an earlier, or a similar, nonconformity reoccurring;

(ii) to reduce the likelihood of an earlier, or a similar, type of patient complaint reoccurring;

(iii) to prevent an untoward event from occurring for the first time, as determined by risk assessments (RAs), or failure mode and effect analysis (FMEAs);

(iv) to prevent an untoward event from occurring for the first time because of a very high consequence rating for a specific possible fault or mistake;

(v) to prevent an untoward event from occurring for the first time because of new knowledge, new technology or new evidence.

Preventive action must always be appropriate to the impact of the problem encountered and the likelihood of it happening again. In the second group of possibilities, (iii)–(iv), in which an event has not yet occurred, any preventive action taken must likewise be commensurate with the perceived likelihood of the untoward incident taking place, but also with the seriousness of the consequences that might occur.

2. Scope

This procedure applies to all types of preventive action taken by the hospital.

3. Responsibilities

It is the responsibility of the quality manager to ensure that all preventive actions are dealt with in an expeditious manner and that appropriate documentation is produced.

4. Associated documents

Procedures:

PC 103 Internal Audit

PC 104 Control of Nonconforming Product

PC 105 Corrective Action

Patient Advisory and Liaison Service (PALS) (see Appendix 3)

Forms:

Nonconformity or Observation Form, FM 124

Nonconformity Form, FM 132

Patient Complaint Form, FM 142

5. Details of procedure

5.1 Preventive actions

Preventive action is essentially a forwards looking phenomenon, starting from the time that a decision is made that corrective action is necessary to put right what is going wrong or has gone wrong.

Preventive action might be taken to prevent a reoccurrence of a nonconformity or a patient complaint.

Preventive action is also taken to prevent an untoward event from occurring for the first time. Such preventive action might be considered necessary in the light of risk assessments and the consequences identified as well as any new evidence, new knowledge or new technology that has led the hospital to believe that an untoward event might happen in the future.

The implementation of the preventive action may not always be possible immediately, but it will take place as soon as possible or practical.

5.2 Nonconformities and patient complaints

5.2.1 Preventive actions and nonconformities

If a decision is taken that there is a need to take preventive action, this should be entered on a nonconformity form, such as an FM 124 or FM 132, as explained in procedures PC 103 (Internal Audit) and PC 104 (Control of Nonconforming Product) respectively. The entry should give the name of the individual responsible for carrying out the preventive action and the date by which it is to be completed.

5.2.2 Preventive actions and patient complaints

Patient complaints are addressed in procedure PC 105 (Corrective Action) and the Patient Complaint Form FM 142 will have been used to record details of the complaint.

If a decision is taken that there is a need to take preventive action, this should be entered on a Patient Complaint Form FM 142. The entry should give the name of the individual responsible for carrying out the preventive action and the date by which it is to be completed.

5.2.3 Verification of any preventive actions arising from nonconformities and patient complaints

In the case of preventive actions arising from nonconformities and patient complaints, the prescribed forms (FM 124, FM 132 and FM 142) should be signed off only by a responsible person within the hospital, usually the quality manager, when they are satisfied that any preventive actions planned have been satisfactorily dealt with from every point of view.

Finally, the preventive action taken should also be reviewed to decide whether the action taken has been effective in dealing with the nonconformity or patient complaint.

5.3 Prevention of future untoward events

5.3.1 Routine planning

Patient safety in hospitals is of paramount importance. Yet there are risks to be faced by many patients in hospitals. For instance, there are risks associated from cross-infections simply from being in or visiting hospital. There are risks from all surgical operations but the risks are usually known and accepted because of the enormous benefits that accrue from such operations. Such risks are insignificant compared with the risks incurred by all of us when outside hospitals from, for instance, road accidents. Nevertheless, top management of a hospital will have documentation in place to minimize the risks involved in a number of areas, including any clinical risks. These will include:

- health and safety policy;
- fire safety policy;
- cross-infection in the hospital.

Such documentation includes standard procedures and actions that should prevent any untoward events, or at worst minimize the effects of untoward events, involving patients and hospital staff. The quality manager is responsible for ensuring that all such documentation is kept up to date in accordance with the latest statutory and legal requirements.

The quality manager is responsible for ensuring that all hospital employees are regularly briefed on the prevention of untoward events and on the documents that are in place for dealing with such events. The personnel department will keep and maintain records of all employees who attend such briefings.

5.3.2 Risk Assessments (RAs): Risk Analysis Numbers

When contemplating future untoward events, it is helpful to make an estimate of the likelihood of it happening and its resulting consequences.

Simple risk analysis is a method of combining both the likelihood and consequences of an untoward event. The risk analysis number is based on two estimated numbers.

Risk Analysis Number = qualitative measure of probability of an untoward event occurring
qualitative measure of the consequences of its occurrence

A qualitative measure of the **probability** of an untoward event occurring can be rated between 1 and 10 as follows:

1. Impossible.
2. Rare. Event will occur only in exceptional circumstances.
4. Unlikely. The event could occur sometime.
6. Moderate. The event will occur at some time.
8. Likely. The event will occur.
10. Certain. The event is expected to occur sometime.

A qualitative measure of the **consequence** of an untoward event occurring might be rated between 1 and 10 as follows:

1. Negligible. No injuries. No financial loss.
2. Minor. First aid treatment. Moderate financial loss.
4. Serious. Medical treatment necessary. High financial implications.
6. Major. Excessive injuries. Major financial loss.
8. Single death.
10. Multiple deaths.

Qualitative risk assessment matrix

Probability		Impossible	Rare	Unlikely	Moderate	Likely	Certain
		1	2	4	6	8	10
Consequence							
Negligible	1	1	2	4	6	8	10
Minor	2	2	4	8	12	16	20
Serious	4	4	8	16	24	32	40
Major	6	6	12	24	36	48	**60**
Death	8	8	16	32	48	**64**	**80**
Deaths	10	10	20	40	**60**	**80**	**100**

The two numbers chosen are multiplied together to give a risk analysis (RA) number. The levels of risk matrix can be established using all possible combinations of numbers. Each number provides an estimate of the probability of an untoward event happening. The higher the number, the more serious the failure mode. The chart clearly indicates that an untoward event has virtually 'no risk' at one extreme and 'high risk' at the other, as shown by the **bold** numbers 60, 64, 80 and 100.

In cases of calculated high risk for an event happening, preventive action is taken to reduce the probability of an untoward event occurring. The high risk numbers should help a hospital to get its priorities right in deciding what preventive actions (not corrective actions) should be addressed.

Although the calculated RA numbers are extremely useful, preventive action, or actions, are also given to any possible causes of failure that have been given a high consequence rating such as 8 or 10.

5.3.3 Other risk management techniques

Other risk management techniques are also available. One such technique is failure mode and effective analysis (FMEA). This is a little more sophisticated than the simple technique referred to above and is based on three estimated numbers, rather than two.

5.3.4 New evidence and new knowledge

Sometimes the possibility of an untoward event can become apparent in the light of new evidence, new knowledge or new technology. Preventive action should be taken to prevent what hitherto was not considered a risk.

5.3.5 Records

All changes arising from preventive actions will be recorded and maintained for future reference.

Appendix 2: Background to clinical governance in hospitals in the UK

Medical audit

Medical audit was recommended by the Department of Health in 1989. In an NHS working paper [10] they defined it as:

> The systematic, critical analysis of the quality of medical care, including the procedures used for diagnosis and treatment, the use of resources, and the resulting outcome and quality of life for the patient.

The paper also adds:

> An effective programme of audit will help to provide the necessary reassurance to doctors, patients and managers that the best possible quality of service is being achieved within the resources available.

However, the purpose of medical audit was seen by the royal colleges as a learning or educational function and not a managerial function, as they emphasized that the outcomes of audits should remain confidential [11].

Clinical audit

In 1993, a multidisciplinary approach was recommended in which medical audit, nursing audit and therapy audit were combined. This multidisciplinary approach was referred to as clinical audit, but there was a significant change with it. Clinical audits were not merely to be educational in nature; they were also intended to engender opportunities for changing clinical practice and thereby improve the quality of service [12].

In the past, clinical audits have not always brought about desirable changes in clinical practice, but the publication of *Principles for Best Practice in Clinical Audit* by NICE [13] should bring about changes in the attitudes of clinical staff to clinical audit. In the foreword to the book, written by Dame Deirdre Hine (Chair of the Commission for Health Improvement) and Professor Sir Michael Rawlins (Chairman of the National Institute for Clinical Excellence) they state that:

> Clinical audit is at the heart of clinical governance.

Corporate governance

Corporate governance is the action, manner or system of controlling a corporate body.

Sir Adrian Cadbury's Committee was set up in May 1991 by the Financial Reporting Council of the London Stock Exchange and the accountancy profession to address the financial aspects of corporate governance following some spectacular corporate failures and frauds. It reported in 1992 on the need for a recommended code of best practice for corporate bodies [2]. The principles on which the code is based are those of openness, integrity and accountability.

> Openness on the part of companies, within the limits set by their competitive position is the basis of all those who have a stake in its success.
>
> Integrity means both straightforward dealing and completeness. What is required of financial reporting is that it should be honest and that it should present a balanced picture of the state of the company's affairs. The integrity of reports depends on the integrity of those who prepare and present them.
>
> Boards of directors are accountable to their shareholders and both have to play their part in making that accountability effective. Boards of directors need to do so through the quality of the information which they provide to shareholders, and shareholders through their willingness to exercise their responsibilities as owners.

The Cadbury report also stressed that non-executive directors should be able to exercise their 'independence of judgement'. Since the publication of the report, the deliberations of other committees have made other recommendations that non-executive directors be given many other specific responsibilities, so much so that being a non-executive director is now more onerous than it was before the Cadbury report [14].

There are critics of corporate governance. One claims:

> There is no evidence that the spreading tentacles of corporate governance have reduced executive remuneration, or had any beneficial effect at all on corporate financial performance or customer satisfaction [15].

Clinical governance: an overview

Clinical governance was first mentioned in an NHS white paper published in 1997 [16]. The purpose of clinical governance was to ensure that quality was at the core of all hospital activities, although the white paper does not explain what was meant by quality. Clinicians (including consultants), nursing staff, managers and all other staff were expected to embrace quality. Nobody was to be excluded.

Clinical governance is defined:

> as a framework through which NHS organizations are accountable for continuously improving the quality of their services and safeguarding high standards of care by creating an environment in which excellence in clinical care will flourish [17].

Clinical governance was generally introduced into NHS hospitals in 1999. Since 1 April 1999, chief executives have had the responsibility not only for financial probity, but also for the quality of care of patients in their hospitals.

Clinical governance is a challenge to all clinicians and all managers. Since the chief executive now must report to the board and to the government on clinical governance, there must be clear lines of responsibility for the overall quality of clinical care.

Each chief executive in consultation with their medical colleagues can decide how clinical governance will be managed. The clinical governance committee of a hospital will consider all aspects of the hospital's work. Membership of the committee will include clinicians, nurses, therapists and many others who support clinicians in their work. Commonly, the clinical governance committee is chaired by the chief executive, director of nursing or the medical director of the NHS Trust.

Clinical governance is about creating an environment in which all clinical professionals are encouraged to improve their clinical and professional performance. With the occurrence of a number of highly publicized failings, such as the Bristol heart scandal, clinical governance became even more important. Clinical governance requires a new culture in which everyone is working for the benefit of patients and everyone can demonstrate their contribution to the system of care.

Traditionally, doctors have always been allowed to do things their own way, justified by their so-called clinical freedom. However, any doctor should realize that their own experience, however great, will inevitably be incomplete as best practice is established from the whole gamut of experiences from doctors who are treating patients with the same or similar diseases or problems. Increasingly, neither health policy nor clinical decisions can any longer be comfortably based on personal opinions and personal experience alone. Fortunately, clinical decisions are gradually becoming more and more 'evidence based' with consequential improvements in the quality of patient care [18]. Evidence-based medicine is a core component of clinical governance. The clinical governance committee should be aiming to develop and enhance clinical practice through the recommendations of NICE and NSFs. By such means, the clinical governance committee will make positive recommendations in the hope that the care of patients in its NHS trust hospital is improved in accordance with the latest information available and that there is therefore continual improvement in the quality of patient care. At the other end of the spectrum, poor practices and poor outcomes should be identified and eliminated.

The collection of relevant data is of paramount importance in the pursuance of clinical governance. This requires careful documentation of each case, done in such a manner that objective evidence can be collected, collated and analysed. Thus, scientifically based outcomes can be generated for comparison with the outcomes for other patients in other hospitals. A renewed commitment to the accuracy, appropriateness, completeness and analysis of health care information is required if correct judgements are to be made about clinical quality, and the validity and impact of clinical governance.

The findings of clinical governance reviews must be fully documented. Reports must be submitted to the chief executive for discussion at board level and subsequently for inclusion in an annual report. When shortcomings are found, steps should be taken to rectify matters. The quality of health care for patients is to be of paramount importance and the safety and protection of patients from untoward events must override all other considerations.

The Commission for Health Improvement, CHI, which began its work on 1 April 2000, is now carrying out independent external clinical governance reviews on every NHS trust and other parts of the NHS. All its reports are in the public domain. This work has now been taken over by CHAI (see Appendix 3).

Appendix 3: Developments in the care of patients in the UK

National Institute for Clinical Excellence (NICE)

The National Institute for Clinical Excellence was established by the government in 1999 as a Special Health Authority and, as such, is part of the National Health Service in England and Wales. It is an independent organization responsible for providing national guidance on treatments and care within the NHS. It promotes clinical excellence and the effective use of resources in the NHS.

The work of NICE comprises three main areas:

- technology appraisals: the use of new and existing medicines and treatments;
- clinical guidelines: the appropriate treatment and care of people with specific diseases and conditions;
- interventional procedures: whether interventional procedures used for diagnosis or treatment are safe and effective enough for routine use.

NICE aims to provide authoritative clear national guidance for all health professionals as part of a process for improving health care. The committee will also review local and national incidents and thereby make recommendations on clinical practice at local level.

The NICE website can be located at www.nice.org.uk.

National Service Frameworks (NSF)

The intention of this initiative is to focus on major conditions such as cardiac disease, cancer and mental health. It will state how these services can be organized in the best way for patients and will identify the standards that have to be reached.

If centres of excellence can be identified in certain hospitals their practices should be considered as a basis for further improvements in other hospitals so that unacceptable variations in performance across the country can be eliminated.

Patient complaints under clinical governance and the Patient Advice and Liaison Services (PALS)

All patient complaints must be taken seriously. Patient complaints might arise from any cause, but occasionally they might arise from a nonconformity. Some complaints, when fully investigated, might prove to be unjustified but it is wise to assume in the first instance that the complaint is justified. Complainants want their views to be acknowledged. They want an explanation for what has occurred (or has not occurred as the case may be). Quite often a simple apology may be all that is needed.

In serious circumstances, the patients, or the relatives of the patient want corrective action to be taken as soon as possible to put right what is going wrong or what has gone wrong. Some might also want to be reassured that action will be taken, preventive action, to reduce the likelihood of a similar occurrence in the future.

In some cases of gross negligence or incompetence of hospital staff, legal action might be instigated to establish all the facts and determine whether financial compensation can be made.

The Wilson Report [19] recommended three principles:

- there should be a common system for complaints covering all NHS services;
- the complaints system should be geared to complainant's concerns and that any disciplinary action should be kept separate;
- there should be a two stage approach: the first in-house, starting where the complaint has arisen; the second an investigation by an independent panel.

At least once each year, hospitals are now required to give information on:

- the number of complaints;
- the type of complaints;
- how quickly complaints were addressed;
- actions taken;
- information passed to top management.

Things go wrong in all organizations because of failings of individuals, management and processes. Risk management decisions can minimize any shortcomings in the delivery of patient care, but they will never entirely eliminate it, hence the importance of addressing all complaints carefully in accordance with the guidelines laid down.

An important aspect of every complaint is to learn from any mistakes made and to ensure that protocols and procedures are in place so that the same mistakes are unlikely to happen in the future.

An NHS Complaints Procedure based on the Wilson recommendations was introduced in 1996. Subsequently, in 1999, the Department of Health commissioned a two-year UK wide evaluation of complaints. Their publication, *Delivering the NHS Plan* [20], includes an annex that summarizes how complaints will be addressed.

Stage 1 – Local resolution

Once a complaint is received it will be processed effectively and efficiently within appropriate time limits.

The board of hospitals should receive (at least quarterly) reports on the causes of complaints and the action taken or proposed to prevent a reoccurrence. The quarterly reports should be submitted to the proposed patients' forums in England for NHS trusts.

Stage 2 – Independent reviews

If a patient is not satisfied with the outcome of a local resolution, they may ask for an independent review. Under present guidelines a convener decides, after consultation with an independent person, if an independent review panel is appropriate. The independent review panel will consist of three members: a lay chairman, the convener and a third lay member. The panel will investigate the complaint and produce a written report.

Stage 3 – Health service ombudsman

If the complainant remains dissatisfied with the response from the NHS, they may refer the matter to the Health Service Commissioner, sometimes referred to as the ombudsman. The ombudsman is independent of both the NHS and the government.

These measures are intended to resolve patient complaints in a systematic manner as quickly as possible. This is particularly important when an organization such as the NHS has captive customers.

A national system was introduced on 1 April 2002 in all NHS hospitals based on the above principles. The Patient Advice and Liaison Services (PALS) will deal with all patient complaints in an effective and timely manner, although times are not specified in PALS. The complaints procedure is integrated into clinical governance. Patients can always resort to common law.

The later report [5] gives further guidance on dealing with patient complaints based on feedback from both patients and staff.

The Commission for Health Improvement (CHI)

The Commission for Health Improvement is an independent national body (covering England and Wales) set up to improve the quality of patient care in the NHS. The commission began its work on 1 April 2000.

Six principles have been adopted that underpin all work that will be conducted by CHI:

1. the patient's experience is at the heart of CHI's work;
2. CHI will be independent, rigorous and fair;
3. CHI's approach is developmental and will support the NHS to continually improve;
4. CHI's work will be based on the best available evidence and focus on improvement;
5. CHI will be open and accessible;
6. CHI will apply the same standards of continual improvement to itself that it expects of others.

CHI will carry out clinical governance reviews by visiting every NHS trust and health authority, which includes primary care groups, local health groups and general practices on a rolling programme. The views of patients and all other stakeholders are included in the clinical governance reviews. Most importantly, the reviews will focus on objective evidence, not on opinions.

The CHI and CHAI multidisciplinary investigative teams will be formed from external resources and these teams will visit hospitals every four years, each investigation taking seven days.

Clinical governance reviews have the following functions:

- to confirm that NICE recommendations, NSF requirements and local protocols and procedures are being followed;
- to collect data for future analysis so that comparisons can be made with data from other centres;
- to determine ways in which continual improvements can be made in the delivery of the service provided.

CHI will also investigate serious failures in the NHS. Requests for investigations can be made by members of the public.

CHI has other worthy responsibilities. It directs the clinical audit programme. Each year it produces a star rating for all NHS organizations. It produces patient and staff surveys and an annual report on the state of the NHS. CHI works with all other organizations at home and a significant number abroad, and is continually reviewing its own work to ensure that all patients receive the best possible clinical care in accordance with best practices and developments in medical science and technology.

All the findings of CHI are published and can be obtained from www.chi.nhs.uk.

The National Patient Safety Agency (NPSA)

Clinical governance requires NHS hospitals to minimize the risks to patients. To this end, at the local level, the general remit of a hospital's risk management committee is to set strategies and systems in place to ensure that there is a safe environment for the care of patients and to ensure there is always effective management of untoward incidents. Hospital risk management committees are expected to have in place arrangements for:

- learning from untoward incidents;
- tackling poor clinical performance of doctors.

At national level, the purpose of the new National Patient Safety Agency (NPSA) is to minimize the risks to patients in NHS hospitals by dissemination of knowledge about untoward incidents. The NPSA is a Special Health Authority for England and Wales. It was created in July 2001 with the prime objective of improving the safety of patient care by learning from untoward incidents with patients. Pilot studies of the proposed reporting system have been conducted with a number of NHS trusts and the system became fully operational within all NHS trusts by the end of 2003 [21].

The idea behind the new agency is that dissemination of untoward clinical experiences (adverse events and near misses) should result in improvements in the quality of health care in our hospitals by enabling clinicians to learn from one another when things go wrong. In some cases, timely clinical intervention can resolve the situation. Such incidents are referred to as near misses. Sadly, in other, cases things go irretrievably wrong with disastrous consequences for a patient. Under this national scheme it will become mandatory for all NHS hospitals to report adverse events and near misses to the agency. The agency will collect and analyse information on such incidents. It will correlate it with any other similar incidents and any relevant information from other sources. Most important of all, it will endeavour to determine the causes of untoward incidents and take appropriate action to prevent them from reoccurring.

In addition, doctors demonstrating evidence of poor clinical performance are expected to be identified early so that any risks to patients can be reduced. This may necessitate reformed professional regulation through changes in the structure and functions of the General Medical Council to ensure enhanced accountability, more transparency, greater involvement of patients and faster, more responsive, procedures to protect patients from the poor clinical performance of doctors.

Serious incidents will continue to be investigated by the local hospitals and independently by the Department of Health or by the Commission for Health Audit and Improvement (CHAI). The agency's task is different: it will record all such events, correlate and analyse the data and identify any trends and reoccurrences with the sole objective of taking appropriate preventive action so that the situation in question does not reoccur.

Although, as stated above, it will be mandatory to report adverse events and near misses to the agency, its work is dependent on a new culture being established in hospitals of openness, integrity and accountability, the key factors required in corporate governance and clinical governance.

The NPSA website can be located at www.npsa.nhs.uk.

National surveys of patient and user experience

Annual national surveys will provide systematic and comparable information on patient and user experiences in NHS hospitals. The surveys will include many things that patients consider important from the quality of food to the quality of clinical care. If a survey shows that a particular hospital is failing in one way or another to give patient satisfaction, then the CHAI could be asked to investigate matters further.

Commission for Healthcare Audit and Inspection (CHAI)

Before April 2004, NHS hospitals could be subjected to two independent inspections, because the work of the health arm of the Audit Commission and the Commission for Health Improvement (CHI) was uncoordinated. The private health care providers were subject to inspections by the National Care Standards Commission (NCSC). All these organizations have played their part in assessing and regulating health care performance.

The new Commission for Healthcare Audit and Inspection (CHAI), launched on 1 April 2004, is the new integrated inspectorate for health care in England. As stated in Chapter 1 it will bring together the work of:

- the former Commission for Health Improvement (CHI);
- the Audit Commission;
- the Mental Health Act Commission (MHAC); and
- the independent health care work of the National Care Standards Commission (NCSC), which includes oversight of private health care.

CHAI will assess the performance of every part of the NHS, and the private sector, so that both will be inspected against the same criteria. Chief executives who fail to carry out auditing based on the recommendations of a Clinical Governance Committee will in due course be presented with impartial objective evidence.

The principal roles of CHAI are:

- inspecting all NHS hospitals;
- licensing private health care provision;
- conducting NHS 'value for money' audits on a national basis;
- validating published performance assessment statistics on the NHS, including waiting list information;
- publishing star ratings for all NHS organizations with the ability to recommend special measures where there are persistent problems;
- publishing reports on the performance of NHS organizations both individually and collectively;
- independent scrutiny of patient complaints;
- publishing an annual report to parliament on national progress on health care and how resources have been used.

The commissioners and the chief inspector have been appointed by the NHS Appointments Commission. The new commission is independent of the NHS and of the government. It will report annually to parliament on the state of the NHS.

Appendix 4:
References

Standards publications

ISO 9001:2000, *Quality Management Systems – Requirements*

Other publications

[1] ISO 9001 and ISO 14001 certificates, 13th Survey (for 2003). Data can be obtained from any ISO member and from the ISO Central Secretariat. ISBN 0 5660 7900 3 (http://www.iso.ch).

[2] The Committee on the Financial Aspects of Corporate Governance (UK). *The Financial Aspects of Corporate Governance* (The 'Cadbury' Report). London: Gee, 1992.

[3] Department of Health. *A First Class Service: Quality in the New NHS* (consultation document). Crown Copyright, 1998.

[4] Green, D. 'A Definition of Quality'. *Qualityworld*. Institute of Quality Assurance, June 2001.

[5] Department of Health. *NHS Complaints Reform: Making Things Right*. Ref: 30765. Crown Copyright, 2003.

[6] Commission for Health Improvement (CHI). *Investigation into the Diagnostic Imaging Services: Barnet and Chase Farm Hospitals NHS Trust*. The Stationary Office, 2002. ISBN 0 11 703190 9.

[7] Department of Health. *Written complaints about hospital and community services, by service area, in England in 2003 and 2004*. Crown copyright, 2005.

[8] Green, D. *ISO 9000 Quality Systems Auditing*. Aldershot: Gower Publishers Ltd, 1997. ISBN 0 5660 7900 3.

[9] Department of Health. *Reforming the NHS Complaints Procedure: a Listening Document*. Crown Copyright, 2001.

[10] Department of Health. *Medical Audit Review of the NHS Working Paper No. 6*. HMSO, 1989.

[11] Royal College of Physicians of London. *Medical Audit: A First Report: What, Why and How?* London: Royal College of Physicians of London, 1989.

[12] Winyard, G., Moores, Y. *Clinical Audit 1994/1995 and Beyond.* Department of Health. HMSO, 1994.

[13] National Institute for Clinical Excellence (NICE). *Principles for Best Practice in Clinical Audit.* Abingdon: Radcliffe Medical Press Ltd, 2002. ISBN 1 85775 976 1.

[14] Rimington, S (2001) *Open Secret: The Autobiography of the former Director-General of MI5.* London: Hutchinson, 2001.

[15] Gaskell, C. 'Power and Responsibility'. *Engineering Management Journal,* June 2002, p.107.

[16] Department of Health. *The New NHS – Modern – Dependable.* The Stationary Office, 1997. ISBN 0 10 138072 0.

[17] Scally, G., Donaldson, L.J. 'Clinical Governance and the Drive for Quality Improvements in the New NHS in England'. *British Medical Journal.* July 1998.

[18] 'Evidence-based Medicine: A New Approach to Teaching the Practice of Medicine'. *The Journal of the American Medical Association* (JAMA). Vol. 268: November, 1992.

[19] Department of Health. *Being Heard: The Report of the Committee on NHS Complaints Procedures chaired by Professor Alan Wilson,* 1994.

[20] Department of Health. *Delivering the NHS Plan: Next steps on investment, next steps on reform.* The Stationary Office, 2002. ISBN 0 10155 032 4.

[21] National Patient Safety Agency. *NPSA Corporate Plan 2003–2006.*